T0093806

Thieme

Supplement to NANDA International Nursing Diagnoses: Definitions and Classification, 2021–2023 (Twelfth Edition)

New things you need to know

T. Heather Herdman, PhD, RN, FNI, FAAN

Camila Takáo Lopes, PhD, RN, FNI

Thieme
New York • Stuttgart • Delhi • Rio de Janeiro

Library of Congress Cataloging-in-Publication Data is available from the publisher.

For information on licensing the NANDA International (NANDA-I) nursing diagnostic system or permission to use it in other works, please e-mail: nanda-i@thieme.com; additional product information can be found by visiting: www.thieme.com/nanda-i.

Thieme Medical Publishers, Inc.
333 Seventh Avenue, 18th Floor
New York, NY 10001, USA
www.thieme.com
+1-800-782-3488
customerservice@thieme.com

Cover design: © Thieme
Cover image source: © Gorodenkoff/stock.adobe.com – stock photo. Posed by models
Typesetting by DiTech Process Solutions, India; typeset using Arbortext.
Printed in the USA by King Printing Co., Inc.
DOI 10.1055/b000000888

ISBN: 978-1-68420-583-7
ISSN: 1943-0728

Also available as an e-book:
eISBN (PDF): 978-1-68420-584-4
eISBN (epub): 978-1-68420-586-8

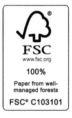

FSC
www.fsc.org
100%
Paper from well-
managed forests
FSC® C103101

Preface

Within the publication of the 12th Edition of the NANDA International, Inc. (NANDA-I) core text, *NANDA International nursing diagnoses: definitions and classification, 2021–2023*, multiple additions, revisions, retirements, and refinements were introduced. The extent of these modifications is a testament to the continued evolution of nursing knowledge and NANDA-I's improved representation of that knowledge within the nursing diagnosis classification.

Please be aware that this companion book is not written to be the primary text for those readers who are new to nursing diagnosis. These individuals should read the text, *NANDA International nursing diagnoses: definitions and classification, 2021–2023*, which includes chapters on the basics of diagnosis, assessment, clinical reasoning and a solid introduction to the NANDA-I taxonomy.

This companion book is designed to give current users of nursing diagnosis a "quick glance" into what is new in the 12th edition, as well as more in-depth information on some of those changes, including the new diagnoses themselves. In addition, conceptual issues that we believe require additional clarification in the upcoming 13th edition will be discussed, and some recommendations will be made for modification as the classification continues to move forward.

We hope that you will find this book helpful as you use nursing diagnosis in your daily practice.

Best wishes,

T. Heather Herdman

Camila Takáo Lopes

Contents

Part 2 Basic understanding of 46 New Nursing Diagnoses

Part 1
NANDA-I Definitions and classification: What is new in the 12th edition?

1   What is new?

1.1 Introduction

As in the previous version, in this chapter you will find the addition of new nursing diagnoses, revisions to existing diagnoses, and retirement of diagnoses from the classification due to an unsatisfactory level of evidence. All of these modifications are introduced in the *NANDA-I nursing diagnoses: definitions and classification, 2021–2023* textbook. However, the purpose of this companion book is to provide more in-depth information to assist your understanding, to support education, and to facilitate implementation of these changes in practice.

1.2 46 New Nursing Diagnoses

NANDA International Nursing Diagnoses: Definitions & Classification, 2021–2023, pp. 24–29. There were 46 new nursing diagnoses in this edition. Each of these diagnoses will be discussed in Part 2 (p. 39), in which we provide a case study for each diagnosis, along with some examples of outcomes and interventions, which are not intended to be a complete list or a definitive plan of care, but rather an example to enhance learning and comprehension.

These will be discussed in detail in Part 2 (p. 39), with model case studies, ultimate goals, outcomes, and nursing actions.

1.3 Revisions to 17 nursing diagnosis labels

NANDA International Nursing Diagnoses: Definitions & Classification, 2021–2023, pp. 37–38. Changes were made to 17 nursing diagnosis labels, as seen in ▶ Table 1.2. Some background was provided on page 37 of the core NANDA-I textbook; however, here we will provide some more detailed explanation.

Changes identified in ▶ Table 1.2 were due to the lack of an identified human response within the label, addition of an axis term to increase specificity of the diagnosis, the need to identify a judgment term within the label, and the need to use terms that describe a concept which are consistent with current conceptual development within the literature.

The following diagnosis labels were changed to ensure a clearly identifiable human response: *ineffective health maintenance, ineffective health management, readiness for enhanced health management, impaired home maintenance, risk for suicide.*

Table 1.1 New nursing diagnoses by domain

Domain	Nursing diagnosis label	Code
1. Health Promotion	Risk for elopement attempt	00290
	Readiness for enhanced exercise engagement	00307
	Ineffective health maintenance behaviors*	00292
	Ineffective health self-management*	00276
	Readiness for enhanced health self-management*	00293
	Ineffective family health self-management*	00294
	Ineffective home maintenance behaviors*	00300
	Risk for ineffective home maintenance behaviors	00308
	Readiness for enhanced home maintenance behaviors	00309
2. Nutrition	Ineffective infant suck-swallow response*	00295
	Risk for metabolic syndrome*	00296
3. Elimination and Exchange	Disability-associated urinary incontinence*	00297
	Mixed urinary incontinence	00310
	Risk for urinary retention	00322
	Impaired bowel continence*	00319
4. Activity / rest	Decreased activity tolerance*	00298
	Risk for decreased activity tolerance*	00299
	Risk for impaired cardiovascular function	00311
	Ineffective lymphedema self-management	00278
	Risk for ineffective lymphedema self-management	00281
	Risk for thrombosis	00291
	Dysfunctional adult ventilatory weaning response	00318
5. Perception / cognition	Disturbed thought process	00279
7. Role relationship	Disturbed family identity syndrome	00283
	Risk for disturbed family identity syndrome	00284
9. Coping / stress tolerance	Maladaptive grieving*	00301
	Risk for maladaptive grieving*	00302
	Readiness for enhanced grieving	00285
11. Safety / protection	Ineffective dry eye self-management	00277
	Risk for adult falls*	00303
	Risk for child falls	00306
	Nipple-areolar complex injury	00320
	Risk for nipple-areolar complex injury	00321
	Adult pressure injury	00312
	Risk for adult pressure injury*	00304

Table 1.1 *continued*

Domain	Nursing diagnosis label	Code
	Child pressure injury	00313
	Risk for child pressure injury	00286
	Neonatal pressure injury	00287
	Risk for neonatal pressure injury	00288
	Risk for suicidal behavior*	00289
	Neonatal hypothermia	00280
	Risk for neonatal hypothermia	00282
13. Growth / development	Delayed child development	00314
	Risk for delayed child development*	00305
	Delayed infant motor development	00315
	Risk for delayed infant motor development	00316

*For taxonomic purposes, when a diagnosis label and definition are revised, the original code is retired and a new code is assigned

In the following labels, an axis term was added to increase the specificity of the diagnosis: *risk for falls, risk for pressure injury, risk for delayed development.*

In the following labels, it was noted that there was an opportunity to identify a judgment term within the label: *bowel incontinence, activity intolerance, risk for activity intolerance.*

Finally, the following labels were changed due to the need to use terms that describe a concept which are consistent with current conceptual development within the literature: *ineffective health management, readiness for enhanced health management, ineffective family health management, ineffective infant feeding pattern, risk for metabolic imbalance syndrome, functional urinary incontinence, complicated grieving, risk for complicated grieving.*

NANDA-I consistently reviews the classification to improve consistency within the terms. If you notice additional areas of inconsistency between terms, we would encourage you to provide feedback for the Diagnosis Development Committee, at: diagnosis@nanda.org.

1.4 Revisions to 67 nursing diagnoses

NANDA International Nursing Diagnoses: Definitions & Classification, 2021–2023, pp. 30–37. Sixty-seven diagnoses were revised during this cycle. Please see the *NANDA International nursing diagnoses: definitions and classification, 2021–2023* textbook for revised definitions and diagnostic indicators

Table 1.2 Changes to nursing diagnosis labels

Domain	Former label	Diagnosis Code	New Label	Diagnosis Code
1. Health promotion	Ineffective health maintenance	00099	Ineffective health maintenance behaviors	00292
	Ineffective health management	00078	Ineffective health self-management	00276
	Readiness for enhanced health management	00162	Readiness for enhanced health self-management	00293
	Ineffective family health management	00080	Ineffective family health self-management	00294
	Impaired home maintenance*	00098	Ineffective home maintenance behaviors	00300
2. Nutrition	Ineffective infant feeding pattern	00107	Ineffective infant suck-swallow response	00295
	Risk for metabolic imbalance syndrome	00263	Risk for metabolic syndrome	00296
3. Elimination and Exchange	Functional urinary incontinence	00020	Disability-associated urinary incontinence	00297
	Bowel incontinence	00014	Impaired bowel continence	00319
4. Activity / rest	Activity intolerance	00092	Decreased activity tolerance	00298
	Risk for activity intolerance	00094	Risk for decreased activity tolerance	00299
9. Coping / stress tolerance	Complicated grieving	00135	Maladaptive grieving	00301
	Risk for complicated grieving	00172	Risk for maladaptive grieving	00302
11. Safety / protection	Risk for falls	00155	Risk for adult falls	00303
	Risk for pressure ulcer	00249	Risk for adult pressure injury	00304
	Risk for suicide	00150	Risk for suicidal behavior	00289
13. Growth / development	Risk for delayed development	00112	Risk for delayed child development	00305

(defining characteristics, related factors, and risk factors) and submitters. Table 1.2 in that book (pp. 31–33) identifies all revisions that were made.

All literature references that were used as evidence to support the submission of these diagnoses are available from the website www.thieme.com/nanda-i.

1.5 23 retired nursing diagnoses

NANDA International Nursing Diagnoses: Definitions & Classification, 2021–2023, pp. 37–41. Twenty-three nursing diagnoses were removed from the classification. Please see the *NANDA International nursing diagnoses: definitions and classification, 2021–2023* textbook for retired diagnoses. Table 1.4 in that book (p. 39) identifies all diagnoses that were removed.

1.6 Standardization of diagnostic indicator terms

NANDA International Nursing Diagnoses: Definitions & Classification, 2021–2023, pp. 41–44. Several minor edits were made to diagnostic indicator terms, or our related factors and defining characteristics (e.g., *alteration in metabolism* was changed to *altered metabolism*). Work was also completed on all associated conditions and at-risk populations to increase clarity and reduce duplication of terms. The editorial changes to these diagnoses should improve translation, improve terminological consistency, and facilitate diagnostic indicator coding.

The editors acknowledge that some of the remaining terms used for diagnostic indicators may be vague or require additional clarification to improve clinical usefulness. What is important in standardizing terms is a definition. The common definition guarantees that nurses can use the term anytime, anywhere, and in the same way. Given this perspective, as each NANDA-I nursing diagnosis has a definition, we may need definitions for diagnostic indicator terms. However, this will be no easy task as there are over 3500 such terms!

We welcome user recommendations in terms of ways to improve these terms to make them more clinically useful.

2 Issues and upcoming activities

In recent versions of the *NANDA-I definitions & classification* textbook, we discussed many issues within the NANDA-I classification. While some of these have been resolved, others remain and require work over the upcoming years.

The evolution of our scientific language is a continual process; there is no "end point" at which the classification will be "complete". Rather, there will be continued revisions, removals from, and additions to the classification as knowledge evolves. Likewise, there are ways to better position the NANDA-I classification as the strongest, most evidence-based, and standardized nursing diagnostic language. Some of these evolutions are more editorial in nature, such as developing a specific schema for definitions and structure of diagnostic indicator terms. Others are more involved, and we will discuss each of these below.

2.1 What is the evidence base for current nursing diagnoses?

Nursing should be an evidence-based science and, as such, requires evidence to support our diagnoses. It is critical that we are able to identify clinical studies that validate nursing diagnoses across populations, cultures, and settings. If differences between the current classification and the clinical study findings are noted, these need to be identified within the classification to ensure support for clinical reasoning.

Many of our current diagnoses are slotted at the lowest level of evidence (LOE) allowed for entry into the classification (2.1). It is believed that, in many cases, these diagnoses actually have significant research findings that would support a higher LOE, but that this work has not been collected and submitted to NANDA-I to enable a higher level of evidence for these diagnoses within the classification. Currently, the NANDA-I Research Committee is conducting many literature reviews to identify potential changes to the LOE. We also look forward to contributions from other nurses interested in such research.

We have numerous diagnoses that were accepted into the classification prior to initiation of LOE criteria, and these require review to determine their LOE status. You might have noticed the following footnote in some diagnoses - *This diagnosis will retire from the NANDA-I classification in the 2024–2026 edition unless additional work is completed to bring it up to a level of evidence 2.1 or higher.* Again, our Research Committee is working on these diagnoses, specifically seeking research evidence to support an accurate, and current, LOE. We hope readers will understand the need to support LOE for all diagnoses, and work with us to advance nursing diagnosis research.

2.2 Can a symptom be a nursing diagnosis?

Although the NANDA-I Taxonomy II uses a multiaxial system, some of the current diagnoses do not fit within this system. They may, in actuality, be symptoms rather than nursing diagnoses, such as: *nausea* (00134), *constipation* (00011), *insomnia* (00095), *fatigue* (00093), *anxiety* (00146), *fear* (00148), *helplessness* (00124), etc. Is the human response we are diagnosing actually *anxiety*, is it the *ineffective management of anxiety*, or is it a *maladaptive threat response*? What is the actual judgment about this symptom/response? Many people experience anxiety at times, and in fact this is a defense mechanism that human beings share; what is the level of anxiety at which this otherwise normal response becomes of concern to nursing?

Currently, we consider *insomnia* and *fear* to be nursing diagnoses, but they can be found as diagnostic indicator terms (defining characteristics/related factors/risk factors) within other nursing diagnoses. Nurses then ask, "Am I supposed to diagnose the *insomnia* itself, or should I consider it as a diagnostic indicator of another nursing diagnosis?" It is difficult to comprehend they can be both defining characteristics and diagnoses. Perhaps instead of *insomnia* we should be considering acute or chronic *deficient sleep,* which is discussed in the literature?

NANDA-I has a team of language developers and taxonomists currently reviewing this issue to determine whether or not symptoms belong within the NANDA-I nursing diagnosis classification. Can we reposition these symptoms within current diagnoses as related factors or defining characteristics? Are there label changes required to represent these concepts? Perhaps a secondary taxonomy of symptoms is needed within NANDA-I, or perhaps we need to determine that these symptoms do not fit within the multiaxial system, and remove them from the classification altogether.

Currently, symptom management is receiving a great deal of attention within the nursing literature. We believe there is a need to reconceptualize symptoms that are found within the NANDA-I taxonomy to reflect this issue. For example, rather than using the diagnosis, *nausea,* perhaps the response is *ineffective nausea management*; rather than *acute pain,* perhaps the response is *ineffective pain management.* However, it would be important that these diagnoses would focus on the client's response, and not an issue with nursing care, as the focus of nursing diagnosis is the client's human response.

2.3 What is the appropriate level of granularity for nursing diagnoses?

One frequent topic of discussion is what level of granularity should be used for diagnoses in the classification. Should the diagnoses be broad, concrete, or both to best support clinical practice? Discussion of levels of granularity is important, because it can support the decision-making of nurses developing/revising diagnoses, and that of those individuals tasked with review of diagnosis submissions to the NANDA-I.

For example, in the most recent NANDA-I release, new diagnoses have been added related to falls, pressure injury, and hypothermia:

- Risk for adult falls (00303)
- Risk for child falls (00306)
- Adult pressure injury (00312)
- Risk for adult pressure injury (00304)
- Child pressure injury (00313)
- Risk for child pressure injury (00286)
- Neonatal pressure injury (00287)
- Risk for neonatal pressure injury (00288)
- Neonatal hypothermia (00280)
- Risk for neonatal hypothermia (00282).

These terms are very specifically diagnosed through assessment data which differ based on the age of the subject, including physiological differences. There are differences in related factors (for example, alcohol consumption is found in *hypothermia* [00007], but delayed breastfeeding is not; the reverse is true in *neonatal hypothermia* [00280]). And, although the defining characteristics are nearly identical in all of the pressure injury diagnoses, differences are found in the related factors as well as the at-risk populations and associated conditions, and these differences can aid diagnosis.

When we look at the foci of diagnoses, we can find different levels of granularity present in the classification. For example, the diagnosis, *risk for hypothermia* (00253) is broader than *risk for neonatal hypothermia* (00282), and *risk for perioperative hypothermia* (00254). Some nurses would argue that *risk for hypothermia* (00253) is the only diagnosis required, because neonatal hypothermia and perioperative hypothermia could be prevented using this diagnosis; other nurses prefer the more concrete diagnoses. In general, however, more granular or more specific diagnoses may better direct specific client care, so long as these diagnoses remain within the domain of independent nursing knowledge and practice.

It is our belief that it is appropriate to have a variety of levels of granularity within the classification. We believe that it is important to have more abstract (broader) terms, because they help us to organize the classification (to classify nursing diagnosis terms). Having the broader term may also support clinical reasoning by helping us to categorize our thinking – you may, for example, notice *risk for infection* (00004) first, and then upon further assessment and/ or reflection, narrow the focus to *risk for surgical site infection* (00266).

However, there would be value in determining what level of granularity would be considered sufficient. For example, considering the examples above, is there a level of granularity that might be considered too discrete? Would we want to have a diagnosis, for example, of *risk for toenail injury*? Would this truly contribute to improved clinical reasoning or change a clinical guideline? These are some of the questions that need to be considered as we continue to grapple with this topic.

2.4 What is needed to improve translation?

The issue of granularity is also important in translation, in the understanding of the focus of the nursing diagnosis in different languages, and in the applicability in clinical practice internationally. An example of this might be the diagnosis, *risk for adult falls* (00303). An individual can fall down the stairs, fall out of bed, or fall down while walking across the room.

However, in the original English language, there is just this one word – "fall" – that is used to express any unintended drop from higher surfaces, or from the same surface. In many languages, this would not be expressed using the same word(s), and so the translation, understanding, and applicability of the original English terms may be difficult. It may be necessary to consider that some languages would be better served to have different nursing diagnosis labels to address those phenomena which cannot accurately be translated as one term from the original English language.

When translating a word in one language to another language, it is often not a one-to-one replacement. For instance, the word "feeding" is included in some diagnoses, such as *feeding self-care deficit* (00102) and *ineffective infant feeding pattern* (00107). In English, the word "feeding" can mean: an instance of eating (e.g., "he is able to manage feeding activities"), *or* taking nourishment (e.g., "the infant is feeding well"), *or* providing nourishment to an individual who is incapable of eating on his own (e.g., "the caregiver is feeding Mr. Jones, who is immobilized after his fall"). In all cases, the English word "feeding" is appropriate and conveys this variety of actions. However, in many languages, these are distinct actions which are discussed using different terms.

Thus, the translation from English into other languages can be confusing and may lose the intended meaning of the term. Back translation may be necessary to ensure that the words used in translation truly match the intent of the original language. Likewise, consideration should be given to determine if there are other words in the original language that would better describe the phenomena and that would be more easily translated. An example of this is our removal of the word "lack" from terms within NANDA-I, after a meeting with the German-speaking network group many years ago, in which we learned that a different word would be used in German to represent "less than" or "none" - both of which are represented in the term "lack" in English. This simple change in the original English text enabled more clarity in translation for the German language, and probably for other languages as well.

Another consideration may be the use of a thesaurus of terms for translation and/or for those terms that are more culturally and clinically relevant. There may be examples in which a term used in English has no actual translation into other languages, and a detailed description is therefore required to facilitate understanding. Matching these descriptions to the original term in a thesaurus ensures that standardization of intent is maintained.

2.5 How should a nursing diagnosis be defined?

In the last three editions, the Diagnosis Development Committee members have worked to bring consistency to the different types of nursing diagnosis definitions. For example, risk and health promotion diagnoses were all changed to reflect similar patterns, respectively. In this manner, risk diagnoses use the format, "Susceptible to…, which may compromise health"; health promotion diagnosis definitions use the phrase "which can be strengthened."

However, some of the definitions of the nursing diagnoses are not particularly helpful to a nurse who is trying to understand the meaning of the diagnoses. For example, it might be helpful for a nurse to see, when looking at the definition of *ineffective health maintenance behaviors* (00292), that the focus of the diagnosis is "health maintenance behaviors", it is located in Class 2 (health management), under Domain 1 (health promotion), and how it is differentiated from other related diagnoses, such as *ineffective health self-management* (00276). This could be accomplished with an outline or mapping of where the concept is located within the taxonomy, along with the verbal description (definition) of the nursing diagnosis itself.

Additionally, some diagnoses adopt definitions that have been approved by national or international groups (e.g., the World Health Organization or the National Pressure Injury Advisory Panel from the USA); in other diagnoses, a definition may be adopted from one particular research article, which is then cited as a reference for the definition; while in others, no particular reference or previously accepted definition is used. No standard currently exists as to when it is appropriate to use a previously accepted definition, when/if one should quote a single article's definition, or if all definitions should be developed specifically for the nursing diagnosis definition within the classification. This issue should be further discussed, until the structure for a diagnosis definition is finalized.

2.6 Syndrome nursing diagnoses

The definition for a syndrome nursing diagnosis indicates that it represents a clinical judgment describing a cluster of nursing diagnoses that occur together, and which are best addressed together and through similar interventions. However, it has not yet been clearly identified whether or not defining characteristics can also include signs/symptoms that are not current nursing diagnoses. Therefore, syndrome diagnoses may currently include nursing diagnoses and other signs/symptoms. This can be confusing to the user, and should be clarified.

We recommend that work be undertaken to remove from the defining characteristics all signs/symptoms that are not represented as nursing diagnoses, or to consider ways to cluster these signs/symptoms together into nursing diagnoses. For example, in the defining characteristics of *relocation stress syndrome* (00114), there are two diagnoses - *anxiety* (00146) and *fear* (00148) - but all others are signs/symptoms. Anxiety and fear are also symptoms, however, as we discussed previously. We need to examine whether "reports altered sleep-wake cycle" is the same as *disturbed sleep pattern* (00198), as well as whether "depressive symptoms", "decreased self concept", "loss of independence", and "low self-esteem" can be replaced with *situational low self-esteem* (00120), for example. We suggest that all syndrome diagnoses should be reviewed and revised to ensure congruence with the definition of syndrome diagnoses.

The other confusing issue for users is when a syndrome is included within a risk nursing diagnosis label. For example, *risk for metabolic imbalance syndrome* (00263) has seven nursing diagnoses listed as risk factors. These diagnoses are risk diagnoses, not syndromes. At present, there is no requirement that risk factors for these syndromes must be nursing diagnoses. The question remains, should the risk factors be nursing diagnoses, or should they be individual symptoms? We suggest that all risk diagnoses which include "syndrome" within the label should be reviewed to establish consistent guidelines for development and use.

2.7 Consistency in use of NANDA-I terms in other works

The purpose of standardization of a classification is to ensure that all nurses can be confident that they understand one another when they communicate their judgments, through the use of the same terms. In other words, if all nurses understand the meaning of a term, such as *decreased activity tolerance* (00298) they will define it in the same way and use the same list of diagnostic indicators to validate their assessment of the phenomena in practice. When this occurs, there is a true standardization of classification. If, however, nurses use the term, *decreased activity intolerance*, but define the phenomena differently or validate it using a different list of indicators, how do we know what is really meant by that term?

To ensure standardization, and the safe use of a classification, NANDA-I began requiring authors to use the exact nursing diagnosis label, definition and diagnostic indicators when using the classification in their own works, beginning with the 9th edition. Authors who adapt, remove or add to the classification must clearly indicate what differs from the NANDA-I terms, as the previous lack of doing so has caused confusion in practice, education and research.

What might appear to be a minor change can, in actuality, have significant implications on the meaning of a term. For example, consider the change of the word "or" to the word "and", in the following definition. *Ineffective breathing pattern* (00032) is defined as the "inspiration and/or expiration that does not provide adequate ventilation." A change in this definition to "inspiration AND expiration..." alters its meaning. Does this now apply to individuals with difficulty with inspiration alone? No, it would not.

Standardization of translations of terms is also a concern. It is important that terms are translated consistently throughout the classification. Further, it is critical that the NANDA-I content is used consistently across other authors' works, and that the official language translations are always used and maintained in their entirety. Again, the purpose here is to avoid confusion and to ensure safety and accuracy in communication.

3   Clinical reasoning models

Clinical reasoning models position nursing diagnosis as the driving force in the nursing process by illustrating logical relationships among nursing diagnosis, outcomes, and interventions. Once a nursing diagnosis is identified accurately, through assessment and based on proper diagnostic indicators (defining characteristics, risk factors, and related factors), you may be surprised by how much easier it is to identify outcomes and select interventions to address the causes and not only the symptoms of a diagnosis. In Part 2 (p. 39), we use these models to identify general goals, outcomes, and nursing actions for the model cases of the 46 new nursing diagnoses.

3.1 Nursing diagnosis drives the nursing process

Without an accurate nursing diagnosis, it is not possible to identify proper nursing outcomes, to plan and implement effective nursing interventions, or to evaluate the progress toward the identified outcomes. In other words, accurate nursing diagnosis is the absolute requirement for the nursing process to flow smoothly. This leads to several questions. How can we identify a nursing diagnosis accurately? How should we identify expected outcomes? How should we select interventions that work for the particular client?

There are some texts which indicate general relationships which exist among the NANDA International (NANDA-I), Nursing Outcomes Classification (NOC), and Nursing Interventions Classification (NIC) (Johnson, et al., 2006) terms. Whether or not these linkages are actually based on sufficient research evidence is unclear, nor are the linkages specified at the etiology level, which is critical. It is also not practical to review these texts for appropriate nursing outcomes and nursing interventions every time we develop a care plan for a nursing diagnosis we have identified. Furthermore, it may take several months, and in some cases several years, after a new edition of NANDA-I classification is released for such books to be published.

Nevertheless, some nurses think that new NANDA-I nursing diagnoses cannot be used until these predefined relationships are available. This is simply not accurate. If standardized nursing language for outcomes or interventions does not exist, or is not in use in one's organization, nurses must clearly document what they intend as an outcome and what interventions they are using to obtain that outcome. Further, each client is unique and so what may be an obvious link in one client will not make sense in another.

There are simple and logical relationships among a nursing diagnosis, outcomes, and nursing interventions. The Clinical Reasoning Model (Kamitsuru, 2009) shows these relationships clearly. A nursing diagnosis plays a role as the driving force of the nursing process. Therefore, once a nursing diagnosis is determined, we simply need to apply basic rules to determine the rest.

The Clinical Reasoning Model was constructed using one of the theory development methods (Kim, 2003). Various authors' perspectives regarding the relationships among nursing diagnosis, nursing outcomes, and nursing interventions were reviewed and deductively synthesized to create the model. The model has been tested at multiple nursing diagnosis workshops, and its usefulness has been confirmed.

The Clinical Reasoning Model consists of three different sub-models:
– Clinical Reasoning Model I: problem-focused nursing diagnosis
– Clinical Reasoning Model II: risk nursing diagnosis
– Clinical Reasoning Model III: health promotion nursing diagnosis.

Each model integrates four essential components of clinical reasoning in the nursing process: diagnostic reasoning, goal and outcome reasoning, nursing intervention reasoning, and evaluation reasoning.

3.2 Clinical reasoning model I: problem-focused nursing diagnosis

Let's start with the model for problem-focused nursing diagnoses (▶ Fig. 3.1). At first glance, the model may seem complicated. However, by breaking it

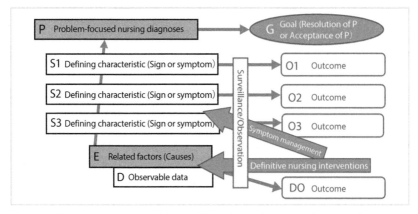

Fig. 3.1 Clinical reasoning model I: problem-focused nursing diagnosis (Reproduced with permission of IGAKU-SHOIN LTD)

down into its four components, it becomes quite simple to understand, and easy to apply in practice.

3.2.1 Problem-focused nursing diagnosis: diagnostic reasoning

▶ Fig. 3.2 shows the *diagnostic reasoning* component. The problem-focused nursing diagnosis consists of:
- P – the label of the nursing diagnosis, problem
- S – the defining characteristics, signs and symptoms
- E – the related factors, etiology, causes of the problem.
- D – the data; if the related factor term is too abstract, it may be helpful to clarify using actual observable data.

Signs are the objective data that the nurse collects through her senses. For example, a client's skin may be dry, smooth, or rough to the touch. The breath sounds may be clear, or there may be rales. *Symptoms* are the subjective data of the client, and what the nurse is told by the client and/or his family/friends. For example, the client may report that he is having trouble with his breathing, or having a sharp pain in his stomach. Signs and symptoms are categorized as *defining characteristics* in the NANDA-I taxonomy.

Related factors are those things that cause or contribute to the diagnosis, and they need either to be modifiable or be able to be removed with independent nursing interventions.

To identify a problem-focused nursing diagnosis accurately, it is important to perform a thorough nursing assessment and identify data and information that support the diagnosis: the defining characteristics and related factors.

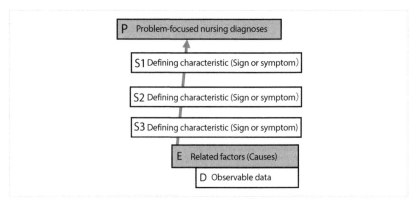

Fig. 3.2 Problem-focused nursing diagnosis: diagnostic reasoning (Reproduced with permission of IGAKU-SHOIN LTD)

Practically, these data and information are collected from the physical examination and interviews.

To identify defining characteristics and related factors to be used as the basis for the diagnosis, please refer to the text, *NANDA International nursing diagnoses: definitions and classification, 2021–2023*. However, some of the diagnoses have a long list of defining characteristics and related factors; and that may be confusing. In such a case, we advise you to review the meaning of the diagnosis by studying the definition, and to utilize your reasoning skills based on accumulated knowledge and experience.

3.2.2 Problem-focused nursing diagnosis: goal and outcome reasoning

The second part of the model is the *goal and outcome reasoning* component (► Fig. 3.3). The goal (G) is at the top right, and it is much broader than outcomes (O). The data outcome (DO) represented in the model is the outcome of the observable data of the related factors.

A goal can either represent the resolution of a problem, or acceptance of the problem. For most of the diagnoses, the goal is resolution of the problem. However, the complete resolution of a chronic problem is not possible, such as with *chronic pain* (00133). In this case, the realistic goal may be acceptance of the problem, followed by strategies to best manage it.

If we view the goal (G) as the ultimate end-point of care, outcomes (O) could be seen as short-term goals or objectives to be achieved as we move toward the ultimate end-point of care. Outcomes are logically derived from the signs and symptoms: the defining characteristics. Likewise, outcomes of

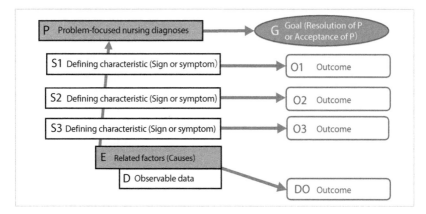

Fig. 3.3 Problem-focused nursing diagnosis: goal and outcome reasoning (Reproduced with permission of IGAKU-SHOIN LTD)

the related factors (causes) can be inferred as the resolution or modification of those factors, and supported by research literature whenever possible.

For instance, goals of the diagnosis, decreased diversional activity engagement (00097) can be easily reasoned from the label; that is, increased diversional activity engagement, or satisfactory diversional activity engagement. If defining characteristics are boredom, frequent naps, and physical deconditioning, then outcomes can be easily reasoned to be reports interest in activities, reports feeling rested, reports feeling alert, and adequate physical conditioning.

Currently different terminologies, such as NOC, are used in conjunction with NANDA-I diagnoses. However, if we adopt validated, standardized scales, we can use them for assessment as well as for evaluation. For example, think about the nursing diagnosis of *adult pressure injury* (00312). If the client has destruction of the skin layers, and this is confirmed objectively using a standardized instrument, then we can use that same scale not only for the daily assessment, but also for evaluating the progress of the skin condition toward identified outcomes. Development of such standardized instruments are an urgent priority for the science of nursing diagnosis.

3.2.3 Problem-focused nursing diagnosis: nursing intervention reasoning

Next is the *nursing intervention reasoning* component (► Fig. 3.4). There are two different arrows pointing from the goal/outcome component. The longer arrow pointing toward the related factors represents the definitive nursing

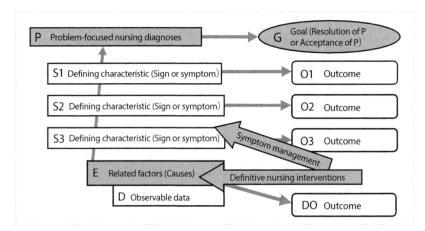

Fig. 3.4 Problem-focused nursing diagnosis: nursing intervention reasoning (Reproduced with permission of IGAKU-SHOIN LTD)

interventions. The other arrow, pointing toward the defining characteristics, relates to symptom management.

Related factors are causes of the problem-focused nursing diagnosis. If we remove those causes through definitive nursing interventions, we can resolve the problem. When defining characteristics include a distressing symptom, symptom management becomes a part of the intervention. *Symptoms* can be treated without treating the cause. By managing symptoms, clients will usually feel ease or relief. Thus, nursing interventions can be logically inferred and selected, using evidence based actions whenever possible, based on the causal related factors and symptoms noted as defining characteristics.

However, in the current NANDA-I classification there are some diagnoses without identified related factors, such as *decreased cardiac output* (00029). With these diagnoses, symptom management becomes the primary nursing intervention.

3.2.4 Problem-focused nursing diagnosis: evaluation reasoning

The last is the *Evaluation reasoning component* (▶ Fig. 3.5). Evaluation in this model reflects ongoing surveillance and observation; in other words, assessment. The rectangular shape representing surveillance and observation is placed between the defining characteristics and the outcomes. What needs to be observed routinely are the four arrows which are covered by the rectangle.

We continuously assess signs and symptoms, used as the basis of the diagnosis, and determine a client's progress toward identified outcomes based on that assessment. We also assess causal related factors and determine how well the client is resolving the underlying cause, as identified in the selected goals.

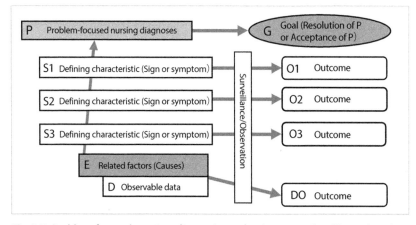

Fig. 3.5 Problem-focused nursing diagnosis: evaluation reasoning (Reproduced with permission of IGAKU-SHOIN LTD)

Through surveillance and observation, we evaluate the effectiveness of nursing interventions. Moreover, we evaluate the improvement of the client's general response (the nursing diagnosis), by evaluating progress toward the identified goal. In addition to those symptoms and signs related to the diagnosis, it is always important to evaluate the general condition of the client, to ensure client safety.

3.2.5 Problem-focused nursing diagnosis: integration

So far, we have explained the model by breaking it down into its four components of clinical reasoning. Let's integrate them by reviewing a client situation (▶ Fig. 3.6).

In this case, we have a client who is exhibiting signs and symptoms of *ineffective airway clearance* (00031), including *ineffective cough, adventitious breath sounds*, and *altered respiratory rhythm*. The causal related factor is *retained secretions*, which is observed as *ineffective sputum elimination*. The established goal seeks to resolve the problem: *clear airway*. Outcomes linked to the signs and symptoms include *effective cough, clear breath sounds*, and *ease of breathing*. Definitive nursing interventions to remove the cause are *hydration* and *coughing instructions*. We continue to assess signs and symptoms, and manifestations of causal factors, to evaluate the effectiveness of nursing interventions. With this client, what we need to assess includes: *cough, breath sounds, respiratory rhythm*, and *amount and characteristics of mucus and sputum*. While assessing these aspects, we can determine the overall condition of the client, *whether he/she has a clear airway*.

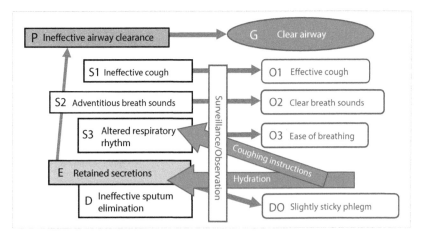

Fig. 3.6 Problem-focused nursing diagnosis: integration (Reproduced with permission of IGAKU-SHOIN LTD)

Here, we have three defining characteristics and one related factor to explain the model as simply as possible. Once the defining characteristics are identified, you need to identify related outcomes. If you find multiple related factors, you need to consider multiple definitive interventions as well as multiple outcomes. Please note that it is NOT our intention to suggest that all nursing diagnoses require three defining characteristics and one related factor: this is simply an example.

3.3 Clinical reasoning model II: risk nursing diagnosis

Now let's examine the clinical reasoning model for risk nursing diagnoses (▶ Fig. 3.7). As with the model for problem-focused nursing diagnosis, we divide the model into four components.

3.3.1 Risk nursing diagnosis: diagnostic reasoning

▶ Fig. 3.8 shows the *diagnostic reasoning* component. The risk nursing diagnosis consists of:
- RP – risk for problem (diagnosis label)
- F – risk factors
- D – observable data; if a risk factor term is too abstract, it may be helpful to clarify using observable data.

To identify a risk nursing diagnosis accurately, it is important to perform a thorough nursing assessment and identify *risk factors*. Risk factors are

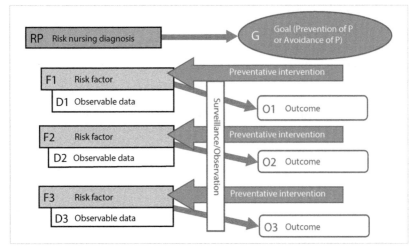

Fig. 3.7 Clinical reasoning model II: risk nursing diagnosis (Reproduced with permission of IGAKU-SHOIN LTD)

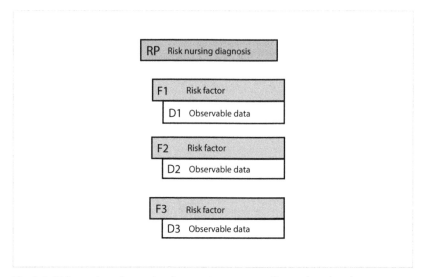

Fig. 3.8 Risk nursing diagnosis: diagnostic reasoning (Reproduced with permission of IGAKU-SHOIN LTD)

environmental factors, and/or physiological, psychological, or chemical elements that increase a client's susceptibility to a response; they can become those things which cause a problem-focused response. In other words, risk factors become related factors when a client's response moves from being a risk nursing diagnosis to a problem-focused nursing diagnosis.

For instance, *imbalance between oxygen supply/demand* is one of the risk factors for the diagnosis, *risk for decreased activity tolerance* (00299). Since we are not able to observe this factor directly, we need to confirm it with observable data, such as *oxygen saturation 92%*, or a client's *report of difficulty breathing during activity*. Risk factors need either to be modifiable or can be eliminated with independent nursing interventions.

3.3.2 Risk nursing diagnosis: goal and outcome reasoning

The second part is the *goal and outcome reasoning* component (▶ Fig. 3.9). The goal (G) is at the top right, and it is always the prevention or avoidance of the problem. Outcomes are generally the resolution or modification of risk factors, and can be logically derived from each risk factor identified.

3.3.3 Risk nursing diagnosis: nursing intervention reasoning

Next is the nursing intervention reasoning component (▶ Fig. 3.10). The three arrows pointing toward the risk factors represent preventative nursing interventions. Preventative nursing interventions are those actions that can remove

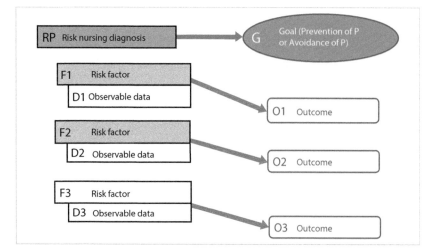

Fig. 3.9 Risk nursing diagnosis: goal and outcome reasoning (Reproduced with permission of IGAKU-SHOIN LTD)

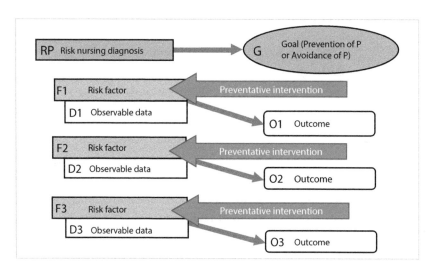

Fig. 3.10 Risk nursing diagnosis: intervention reasoning (Reproduced with permission of IGAKU-SHOIN LTD)

or modify risk factors, in order to prevent or delay a problem from occurring. Thus, nursing interventions for risk nursing diagnosis can be inferred and selected based on the risk factors identified, and supported by research literature whenever possible.

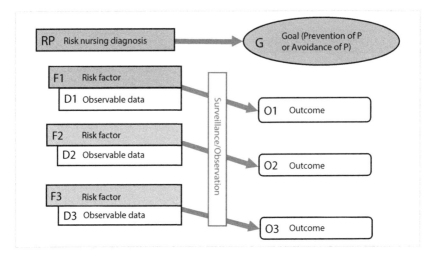

Fig. 3.11 Risk nursing diagnosis: evaluation reasoning (Reproduced with permission of IGAKU-SHOIN LTD)

3.3.4 Risk nursing diagnosis: evaluation reasoning

The last part of the model is the *evaluation reasoning* component (▶ Fig. 3.11). Evaluation in this model requires ongoing surveillance and observations, which again means assessment. Evaluation determines the effectiveness of the preventative nursing interventions that have been implemented. It is also important to evaluate any changes in the condition of the client.

The rectangular shape representing surveillance and observation is placed between the risk factors and the outcomes. What needs to be observed routinely are represented by the three arrows that are covered by the rectangle. We need to assess those risk factors used as the basis of the diagnosis, and determine the client's progress toward resolving those risk factors, as identified by the outcomes.

3.3.5 Risk nursing diagnosis: integration

We have explained the model for risk nursing diagnosis by breaking it down into its four clinical reasoning components. Let's integrate them by reviewing a case (▶ Fig. 3.12).

In this case, we have a caregiver who has three risk factors identified for *risk for caregiver role strain* (00062), including observations of: *social isolation,* as there is *no one with whom she can talk; ineffective coping strategies,* as she has *no effective way to release stress;* and *inadequate respite for caregiver,* because there is *no supportive backup person living nearby.* Based on the

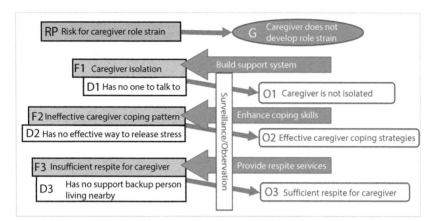

Fig. 3.12 Risk nursing diagnosis: integration (Reproduced with permission of IGAKU-SHOIN LTD)

diagnosis label, we identify a goal: *does not develop caregiver role strain*. In addition, based on the risk factors we can also identify outcomes: *caregiver is not isolated, effective caregiver coping strategies*, and *sufficient respite for caregiver*. Preventative interventions to modify risk factors include: *build support systems, enhance coping skills*, and *provide respite services*. We continue to evaluate the improvement of risk factors to determine the effectiveness of our interventions. What we need to assess includes: *whether or not the caregiver is isolated, whether stress is released effectively*, and *whether the caregiver uses respite when needed*. While assessing these aspects, we determine the overall condition of the caregiver, and *whether the caregiver is free from role strain*.

Finally, we will examine the model for health promotion nursing diagnoses (▶ Fig. 3.13). Here again, we divide the model into four components.

3.4 Clinical reasoning model III: health promotion nursing diagnosis

3.4.1 Health promotion nursing diagnosis: diagnostic reasoning

▶ Fig. 3.14 shows the *diagnostic reasoning* component. A health promotion nursing diagnosis requires:

- HE – health enhancement, (the diagnosis label).
- S – motivation/desire, (defining characteristics).

The health promotion nursing diagnosis is identified based on the expression of the client concerning motivation and desire to increase well-being and to actualize health potential. Therefore, defining characteristics represent such

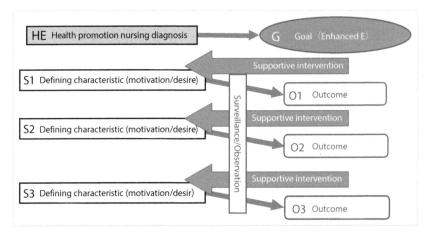

Fig. 3.13 Clinical reasoning model: health promotion nursing diagnosis (Reproduced with permission of IGAKU-SHOIN LTD)

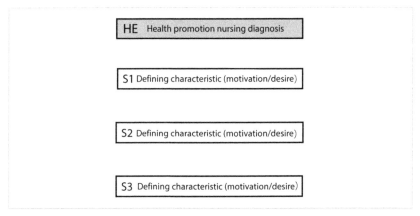

Fig. 3.14 Health promotion nursing diagnosis: diagnostic reasoning (Reproduced
with permission of IGAKU-SHOIN LTD)

statements from the client. To identify a health promotion nursing diagnosis
accurately, it is important to perform a thorough nursing assessment and recognize such statements from the client. If the client is unable to express his/
her desire, the nurse may advocate for health promotion on the client's behalf.

3.4.2 Health promotion nursing diagnosis: goal and outcome
reasoning

The second part is the *goal and outcome reasoning* component (▶ Fig. 3.15).
The final goal (G), is at the top right, and it generally represents an enhancement of the focus of the diagnosis. Outcomes are commonly the attainment of

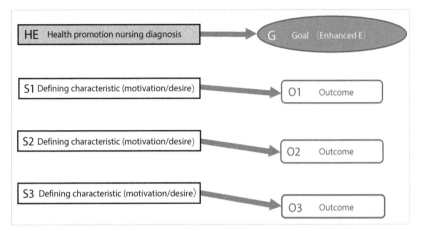

Fig. 3.15 Health promotion nursing diagnosis: goal and outcome reasoning (Reproduced with permission of IGAKU-SHOIN LTD)

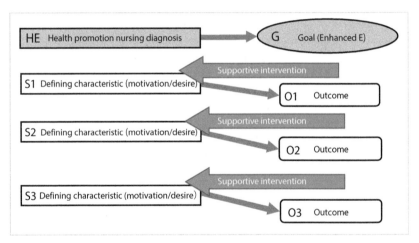

Fig. 3.16 Health promotion nursing diagnosis: nursing intervention reasoning (Reproduced with permission of IGAKU-SHOIN LTD)

whatever health behavior the client desires. Each outcome is logically derived from each defining characteristic.

3.4.3 Health promotion nursing diagnosis: nursing intervention reasoning

Next is the *nursing intervention reasoning* component (▶ Fig. 3.16). The three arrows that point toward the defining characteristics represent supportive nursing interventions. Supportive nursing interventions mean those actions that assist the client in his/her progress towards the identified outcome, while

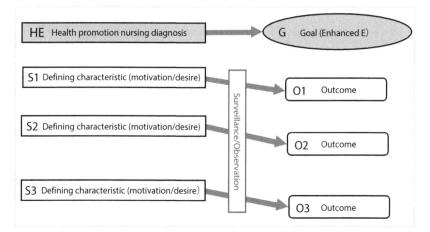

Fig. 3.17 Health promotion nursing diagnosis: evaluation reasoning (Reproduced with permission of IGAKU-SHOIN LTD)

maximizing his/her motivation and desire. Thus, nursing interventions for the diagnosis are inferred and selected based on the confirmed defining characteristics, and supported by research literature whenever possible.

3.4.4 Health promotion nursing diagnosis: evaluation reasoning

The last part of the model is the *evaluation reasoning component* (▶ Fig. 3.17). Evaluation in this model is based on ongoing surveillance and observation; in other words, assessment. Evaluation determines the effectiveness of the supportive nursing interventions that have been implemented.

The rectangular shape representing surveillance and observation is placed between defining characteristics and the outcomes. What needs to be observed routinely are those three arrows that are covered by the rectangle. We need to assess those defining characteristics used as the basis of the diagnosis, and determine the client's progress toward outcomes: the attainment of the health behavior that the client desires.

As we explained in Chapter 2, sometimes the client verbalizes motivation and desire, but makes no progress toward his/her goal. In such a case, it is necessary to discontinue the health promotion nursing diagnosis and consider changing the diagnosis to a risk or problem-focused nursing diagnosis.

3.4.5 Health promotion nursing diagnosis: integration

We explained the model for health promotion nursing diagnosis by breaking it down into its four components of clinical reasoning. Let's integrate these components by reviewing a client situation (▶ Fig. 3.18).

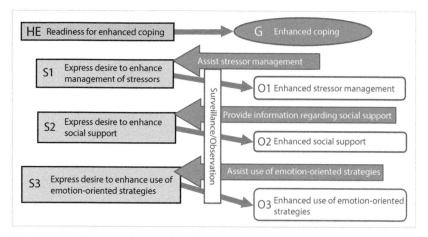

Fig. 3.18 Health promotion nursing diagnosis: integration (Reproduced with permission of IGAKU-SHOIN LTD)

Our case is a new employee who is under various stressors at the workplace. He comes to see the occupational health nurse and reports that he is not feeling well. At first, the nurse considers the problem-focused nursing diagnosis, *ineffective coping* (00069), but he expresses a desire to enhance *management of stressors, social support,* and *use of emotion-oriented strategies.* Since he is clearly expressing these desires, the nurse identifies the health promotion nursing diagnosis, *readiness for enhanced coping* (00158). The nurse identifies the goal, *enhanced coping,* from the label of the diagnosis. Outcomes identified by linking defining characteristics of the diagnosis include: *enhanced stressor management, enhanced social support,* and *enhanced use of emotion-oriented strategies.* Supportive nursing interventions are aimed at the defining characteristics, which include: *assist with stressor management; provide information regarding social support;* and *assist with the use of emotion-oriented strategies.* The nurse continues to evaluate the attainment of the health behavior that he desires, which includes: *management of stressors, social support,* and *use of emotion-oriented strategies.* While assessing these aspects, the nurse determines the overall coping of this employee, or *whether his coping is enhanced.*

Part 2
Basic understanding of 46 New Nursing Diagnoses

Forty-six new diagnoses were approved by the NANDA-I membership (Herdman, Kamitsuru, & Takao Lopes, 2021, pp. 24–29, Table 1.1). On the pages that follow, we provide model cases, key goals and outcomes, and general interventions for these diagnoses to support their use in education, research and practice. Because these are new nursing diagnoses, work is now needed to identify evidence-based outcomes and interventions. Therefore, in this book we are only providing general guidelines with regard to outcomes and interventions.

Please see the *NANDA International Nursing Diagnoses: Definitions and Classification, 2021–2023* textbook for diagnostic indicators (defining characteristics, related factors, risk factors) and submitters. All references that were used with the submission of these diagnoses are available from the website http://www.thieme.com/nanda-i.

Domain 1.
Health promotion

Class 2. Health management
Identifying, controlling, performing, and integrating activities to maintain health and well-being

Code	Diagnosis	Page
00290	Risk for elopement attempt	42
00307	Readiness for enhanced exercise engagement	44
00292	Ineffective health maintenance behaviors	46
00276	Ineffective health self-management	49
00293	Readiness for enhanced health self-management	52
00294	Ineffective family health self-management	54
00300	Ineffective home maintenance behaviors	58
00308	Risk for ineffective home maintenance behaviors	61
00309	Readiness for enhanced home maintenance behaviors	63

Domain 1 • Class 2 • Diagnosis Code 00290

Risk for elopement attempt

Camila Takáo Lopes, Vanessa Ribeiro Neves

NANDA International, Inc. Nursing Diagnoses: Definitions and Classification 2021–2023, 12th Edition, p. 192

Definition
Susceptible to leaving a health care facility or a designated area against recommendation or without communicating to health care professionals or caregivers, which may compromise safety and/or health.

Model case
Mrs. P.L. has been homeless for five years. She was admitted to the emergency room of a public hospital four days ago due to vomiting and renal colic induced by a large stone. Laboratory studies were performed, but she had to wait two days for a computerized tomography (CT) scan because the machine was broken. While waiting for the CT scan, she became very anxious and agitated and left the emergency room without telling anyone. She was readmitted two hours later because her pain had become severe again and she couldn't stop vomiting. Following imaging studies, she underwent a left percutaneous nephrolithotomy. She is now in the immediate postoperative period in the urology unit and has a nephrostomy tube with bloody urine drainage. She is expected to be discharged after 48 hours and will have an ambulatory follow-up evaluation after six weeks, if there are no complications. The social service department at the hospital is involved in arrangements for discharge. However, she has been frequently requesting immediate discharge and walking near the exit door. She has been telling other clients, "they take too long to treat us in this hospital, I don't know why they are keeping us here". She is autopsychically and allopsychically oriented, with periods of allopsychic disorientation.

Assessment
During the assessment, the nurse collected the following data, which could be interpreted to be risk (causative/predisposing) factors for this diagnosis:
- Exit-seeking behavior
- Perceived lack of safety in surrounding environment
- Dissatisfaction with current situation

Although nurses cannot independently intervene upon at risk populations or associated conditions, it is important to be aware of individuals for whom a nursing diagnosis might be more likely to occur. Thus, the nurse should have

identified the following at risk populations that would potentially alert the nurse to concerns for this diagnosis:
- Homeless individuals
- Individuals frequently requesting discharge
- Individuals with history of elopement
- Individuals with impaired judgment

Listed below are some examples of nursing goals, outcomes and actions, linked to etiological factors. This is not presented as a comprehensive plan of care, but rather provides examples to demonstrate the proper method for linking diagnosis to outcomes and interventions, in an evidence-based manner.

Mrs. P.L.'s nursing diagnosis, ultimate goal and outcomes, and general nursing actions

Nursing diagnosis	Risk for elopement attempt (00290)	
Ultimate goal(s)	Absence of elopement attempt	
Risk factors	Outcomes	Nursing actions
Exit-seeking behavior	Remains on unit until discharge	Maintain close and frequent surveillance of unit exit Identify client with elopement risk with institutional bracelet (coded, special color, etc.) Alert unit staff of client's risk for elopement attempt
Perceived lack of safety in surrounding environment Dissatisfaction with current situation	Perceived safety in surrounding environment	Demonstrate empathy regarding feelings Educate on misconceptions about the surgical recovery period Educate on risks of nephrostomy-related complications (e.g. bleeding, infection) Educate on need for professional observation in the 48 hours following surgery Introduce client to each healthcare provider Ensure that procedures are understood before performing them Maintain frequent assessment of orientation status

Domain 1 • Class 2 • Diagnosis Code 00307

Readiness for enhanced exercise engagement

Camila Takáo Lopes, Agueda Maria Ruiz Zimmer Cavalcante

NANDA International, Inc. Nursing Diagnoses: Definitions and Classification 2021–2023, 12th Edition, p. 196

Definition
A pattern of attention to physical activity characterized by planned, structured, repetitive body movements, which can be strengthened.

Model case
Mr. F.D., 52 years old, has hypertension and a family history of cardiovascular disease. His father died at 49, and one of his two brothers died at 52 years of age, both from acute myocardial infarction. Following his brother's death, Mr. F.D's pregnant daughter and wife had a long conversation with him, during which they expressed concerns about his health, especially about his sedentary habits. He agreed to work towards a new lifestyle routine to include physical activity. He expresses the hope to feel less tired and to increase his future capacity to actively engage and play with his grandchild. He tells the nurse he would like to learn about group opportunities in his neighborhood because he would not like to start physical activities by himself.

Assessment
During the assessment, the nurse collected the following data, which would be interpreted as defining characteristics of motivation and desire to increase well-being and to actualize health potential:
- Expresses desire to enhance knowledge about group opportunities or participation in physical activity
- Expresses desire to enhance physical conditioning
- Expresses desire to maintain physical well-being through physical activity
- Expresses desire to meet others' expectations about physical activity plans

Listed below are some examples of nursing goals, outcomes and actions. This is not presented as a comprehensive plan of care, but rather provides examples to demonstrate the proper method for linking diagnosis to outcomes and interventions, in an evidence-based manner.

Mr. F.D.'s nursing diagnosis, ultimate goal, outcomes, and nursing actions

Nursing diagnosis	Readiness for enhanced exercise engagement (00307)	
Ultimate goal(s)	Enhanced exercise engagement	
Defining characteristics	Outcomes	Nursing actions
Expresses desire to enhance knowledge about group opportunities for participation in physical activity	Enhanced knowledge about group opportunities	Provide information on different community resources for group physical activity Provide information on connecting with virtual community groups with similar needs and interests
Expresses desire to enhance physical conditioning	Enhanced physical conditioning	Encourage to determine mid-range goals according to tolerance, starting with a reasonable short-term goal
Expresses desire to maintain physical well-being through physical activity	Physical well-being	Encourage performance of light to moderate exercise for 30 minutes or more on most days of the week Educate to self-monitor progress on physical conditioning and physical well-being Incorporate regular supervision, feedback, and reinforcement strategies Clarify that it is normal to deviate episodically from goal behavior and educate on use of behavioral and cognitive strategies to manage these situations
Expresses desire to meet others' expectations about physical activity plans	Meets expectations about physical activity plans	Emphasize the benefits of physical activity Support commitment to follow plan using short, mid-range, and long-term goals Reinforce importance of maintaining physical activity through consistent motivational messaging Incorporate regular supervision, feedback, and reinforcement strategies

1. Health promotion

Domain 1 • Class 2 • Diagnosis Code 00292

Ineffective health maintenance behaviors

T. Heather Herdman

NANDA International, Inc. Nursing Diagnoses: Definitions and Classification 2021–2023, 12th Edition, p. 199

> **Definition**
> Management of health knowledge, attitudes, and practices underlying health actions that is unsatisfactory for maintaining or improving well-being, or preventing illness and injury.

Model case

Ms. L.P., 32 years old, is obese and has Type 2 Diabetes mellitus, hypertension, and needs a knee replacement. She receives public assistance funds for support and health care, and works part time as a grocery store cashier because she cannot tolerate more than 3 days/week on her feet. She lives alone, has few social connections, and has been frequently hospitalized for depression. She often misses scheduled health care appointments, and indicates that she doesn't trust her providers because they dislike obese individuals and think she deserves to be in pain because of her lifestyle choices.

She has agreed to multiple health plans of action to reduce her risk factors for hypertension and worsening diabetes, and to reduce her weight, but she has repeatedly failed to follow through on these plans. When the nurse asks her to discuss ways to lower her HgbA1C levels and her blood pressure, she refuses to engage in the discussion, indicates she does the best she can do, and just wants to live her life without people telling her what to do.

Assessment

During the assessment, the nurse collected the following data, which could be interpreted to be related (causative) factors for this diagnosis:
- Depressive symptoms
- Inadequate social support
- Inadequate trust in health care professionals
- Perceived prejudice

The nurse also collected the following data, which would be interpreted as defining characteristics for this diagnosis:
- Failure to take action that prevents health problem
- Failure to take action that reduces risk factor
- Inadequate commitment to a plan of action

- Inadequate interest in improving health
- Pattern of lack of health-seeking behavior

Although nurses cannot independently intervene upon at risk populations or associated conditions, it is important to be aware of individuals for whom a nursing diagnosis might be more likely to occur. Thus, the nurse should have identified the following at risk population and associated condition that would potentially alert the nurse to concerns for this diagnosis:

- Economically disadvantaged individuals
- Chronic disease

Listed below are some examples of nursing goals, outcomes and actions, primarily linked to etiological factors. This is not presented as a comprehensive plan of care, but rather provides examples to demonstrate the proper method for linking diagnosis to outcomes and interventions, in an evidence-based manner.

Ms. L.P.'s nursing diagnosis, ultimate goal, outcomes, and nursing actions

Nursing diagnosis	Ineffective health maintenance behaviors (00292)	
Ultimate goal(s)	Effective health maintenance behaviors	
Related factors	Outcomes	Nursing actions
Depressive symptoms	Stabilized mood	Demonstrate acceptance and understanding of depressive symptoms Provide a nonjudgmental approach while preserving confidentiality Monitor severity of depressive symptoms using a standardized tool Let client know that you are concerned and that her feelings matter Refer to specialized psychological care, as needed
Inadequate social support	Adequate social support	Identify and include sources of social support
Inadequate trust in health care professionals	Adequate trust in health care professionals	Assist in identifying peer support group who might assist with self-care Identify and provide information on support groups providing local or online support to individuals with chronic disease Provide in-home, nurse-delivered and culturally sensitive education and home visit intervention targeting Type 2 DM symptom management Provide adherence counseling Provide self-care support Provide stability and consistency in nursing caregivers to enable relationship building and establish trust

Perceived prejudice	Perceive fairness	Encourage sharing of feelings and concerns
		Acknowledge feelings and concerns
		Provide stability and consistency in nursing caregivers to enable relationship building and establish trust
		Provide a non-judgmental approach
		Use silence and active listening during interactions

Domain 1 • Class 2 • Diagnosis Code 00276

Ineffective health self-management

Paula Hino, Anneliese Domingues Wysocki, Camila Takáo Lopes

NANDA International, Inc. Nursing Diagnoses: Definitions and Classification 2021–2023, 12th Edition, p. 201

Definition
Unsatisfactory management of symptoms, treatment regimen, physical, psychosocial, and spiritual consequences and lifestyle changes inherent in living with a chronic condition

Model case
Mr. F.F.J., 41 years old, married, father of three, works night shifts in a 24-hour supermarket from 7 p.m. to 7 a.m. For approximately one month, he has complained of coughing up phlegm, chest pain, lack of appetite, and feeling feverish at the end of the day, which makes him sweat profusely. He noticed that he had been losing weight, because his clothes no longer fit the same. After much insistence from his wife, he sought care from the clinic and the nurse informed Mr. F.F.J. and his wife that his sputum test indicated pulmonary tuberculosis. She provided an explanation about the disease, the recommended directly observed therapy (DOT) for at least six months, and the possible adverse effects of the treatment regimen. She emphasized the importance of starting treatment as soon as possible and completing it, in addition to tracing contacts and screening them for tuberculosis. In the following weeks, Mr. F.F.J. was on a medical leave, so he attended the scheduled DOT daily at 8:30 a.m. at the basic healthcare unit. The nurse later realized that he had attended the scheduled DOT for 16 days only and had missed the following 12 days. She decided to pay him a home visit to investigate what had happened. She found Mr. F.F.J. coughing up phlegm again, experiencing chest pain, fatigue, and increased sweating.

He reports that his symptoms had improved during the two weeks after diagnosis, but now he feels discouraged, as he considers his physical and mental health to be poor, and he cannot even perform leisure activities. He told the nurse that he had been on medical leave for 14 days after his diagnosis, so he had no problems being at the clinic at 8:30 a.m. However, when he returned to his night shift routine, he had to leave his workplace at 7 a.m. and go straight to the clinic. He usually arrived at 7:50 a.m., but he had to wait until 8:30 a.m. for his DOT. He did that for two days, but then he gave up and even missed his follow-up medical appointment because some of his work colleagues convinced him that his disease could not be that serious, that he was probably cured, as he was no longer coughing up phlegm, and that he could just take a home remedy.

Assessment

During the assessment, the nurse collected the following data, which could be interpreted to be related (causative) factors for this diagnosis:

- Perceived barrier to treatment regimen
- Unrealistic perception of seriousness of condition
- Unrealistic perception of treatment benefit

The nurse also collected the following data, which would be interpreted as defining characteristics for this diagnosis:

- Failure to include treatment regimen into daily living
- Failure to attend appointments with health care provider
- Exacerbation of disease signs
- Exacerbation of disease symptoms
- Decreased perceived quality of life

Listed below are some examples of nursing goals, outcomes and actions, primarily linked to etiological factors. This is not presented as a comprehensive plan of care, but rather provides examples to demonstrate the proper method for linking diagnosis to outcomes and interventions, in an evidence-based manner.

Mr. F.F.J.'s nursing diagnosis, ultimate goal, outcomes, and general interventions

Nursing diagnosis	Ineffective health self-management (00276)	
Ultimate goal(s)	Effective health self-management	
Related factors	**Outcomes**	**Nursing actions**
Perceived barrier to treatment regimen	Ability to cope with perceived barrier	Ensure flexibility of care delivery hours for those under directly observed treatment in the clinic
Unrealistic perception of seriousness of condition	Realistic perception of seriousness of condition	Explain and illustrate seriousness of condition Enable access to health care providers to discuss misinformation from others
Unrealistic perception of treatment benefit	Realistic perception of treatment benefit	Discuss benefits of indicated treatment
Defining characteristics	**Outcomes**	**Nursing actions**
Failure to include treatment regimen into daily living	Inclusion of treatment regimen into daily living	Discuss client's co-responsibility in treatment management Discuss potential lack of benefits or harms of unproven methods of treatment Enable access to health care providers to discuss misinformation from others
Failure to attend appointments with health care provider	Attendance at appointments with health care provider	
Exacerbation of disease signs	Absence of disease signs Improved disease signs	Educate on self-monitoring of disease signs Monitor disease signs

Exacerbation of disease symptoms	Absence of disease symptoms Improved disease symptoms	Educate on self-monitoring of disease symptoms Monitor severity of disease symptoms
Decreased perceived quality of life	Improved perceived quality of life	Monitor perceived quality of life using a standardized, validated tool

1. Health promotion

Domain 1 • Class 2 • Diagnosis Code 00293

Readiness for enhanced health self-management

Anneliese Domingues Wysocki, Hugo Fernandes, Camila Takáo Lopes

NANDA International, Inc. Nursing Diagnoses: Definitions and Classification 2021–2023, 12th Edition, p. 203

Definition
A pattern of satisfactory management of symptoms, treatment regimen, physical, psychosocial, and spiritual consequences and lifestyle changes inherent in living with a chronic condition, which can be strengthened.

Model case
Mr. F.F.J., 41 years old, was diagnosed with pulmonary tuberculosis months ago. He and his family had a hard time managing his treatment, symptoms, physical, psychosocial, and spiritual consequences and lifestyle changes. They were diagnosed with *ineffective health self-management* (00276) and *ineffective family health self-management* (00294) by primary healthcare nurses. During the course of treatment for both nursing diagnoses, F.F.J. reports he wished none of this had happened, and says that he really wants to attend his clinic appointments and have medication supervision this time. He expresses wanting to get rid of his coughing and fatigue and gain the weight he lost, so that his work life and social life can go back to normal. He wants to be able to get back to work and talk to his colleagues, have a peaceful home as it used to be with his wife, children and relatives.

Assessment
During the assessment, the nurse collected the following data, which would be interpreted as defining characteristics of motivation and desire to increase well-being and to actualize health potential:
- Expresses desire to enhance commitment to follow-up care
- Expresses desire to enhance inclusion of treatment regimen into daily living
- Expresses desire to enhance management of signs
- Expresses desire to enhance management of symptoms
- Expresses desire to enhance inclusion of treatment regimen into daily living
- Expresses desire to enhance management of signs
- Expresses desire to enhance management of symptoms
- Expresses desire to enhance satisfaction with quality of life

Listed below are some examples of nursing goals, outcomes and actions. This is not presented as a comprehensive plan of care, but rather provides examples to demonstrate the proper method for linking diagnosis to outcomes and interventions, in an evidence-based manner.

Mr. F.F.J.'s nursing diagnosis, ultimate goal, outcomes and nursing actions

Nursing diagnosis	Readiness for enhanced health self-management (00293)	
Ultimate goal(s)	Enhanced health self-management	
Defining characteristics	Outcomes	Nursing actions
Expresses desire to enhance commitment to follow-up care	Enhanced commitment to follow-up care	Encourage commitment to follow-up care on a regular basis
Expresses desire to enhance inclusion of treatment regimen into daily living	Enhanced inclusion of treatment regimen into daily living	Support inclusion of treatment regimen into daily living
Expresses desire to enhance management of signs	Enhanced management of signs	Support with management of signs on a regular basis
Expresses desire to enhance management of symptoms	Enhanced management of symptoms	Support with management of symptoms on a regular basis
Expresses desire to enhance satisfaction with quality of life	Enhanced satisfaction with quality of life	Assess for areas in which client expresses an opportunity for growth Measure satisfaction with quality of life using a standardized, validated tool

1. Health promotion

53

Domain 1 • Class 2 • Diagnosis Code 00294

Ineffective family health self-management

Hugo Fernandes, Paula Hino, Camila Takáo Lopes

NANDA International, Inc. Nursing Diagnoses: Definitions and Classification 2021–2023, 12th Edition, p. 204

Definition
Unsatisfactory management of symptoms, treatment regimen, physical, psychosocial, and spiritual consequences and lifestyle changes inherent in living with one or more family members' chronic condition.

Model case
Mr. F.F.J., 41 years old, was diagnosed with pulmonary tuberculosis months ago. Initially, he followed the directly observed treatment, but lately he has not been adhering fully to treatment, has begun coughing again and presents with lack of appetite and chest pain. He lives in a single-bedroom house, where he sleeps with his wife and their baby son, while their two older children sleep in the living room. The demands from raising three children leave little time for attention to the couple's health needs, especially Mr. F.F.J.'s. There are frequent conflicts between the couple. His wife claims that tuberculosis is God's punishment because of F.F.J.'s lack of commitment to their family and their children's education. She believes that F.F.J. cannot feel so bad that he cannot work every night. In addition, she believes that the recommended treatment has made his health worse, therefore she has been encouraging F.F.J. to stop taking his medication. Their oldest son, aged 11, reports dissatisfaction with his current quality of life, after he told his school friends that his father had tuberculosis, they have been staying away from him and will not play with him or do school activities together. F.F.J.'s mother-in-law and uncles stopped visiting them since they learned that he has tuberculosis. In one of their rare visits, his mother-in-law demanded that he remained in his room while she played with her grandchildren.

In addition, she strongly recommended that F.F.J.'s wife separate his cutlery and utensils from everyone else's in the house. F.F.J.'s wife says she doesn't quite understand this disease, so she immediately accepted her mother's suggestion. She told her mother that she intends to seek professional help because she constantly feels tense, distressed, tearful, and thinks she is depressed. She had never imagined she would have to take care of her husband, in addition to her three children.

Assessment

During the assessment, the nurse collected the following data, which could be interpreted to be related (causative) factors for this diagnosis:

– Competing demands on family unit
– Conflict between spiritual beliefs and treatment regimen
– Difficulty dealing with role changes associated with condition
– Family conflict
– Unsupportive family relations
– Inadequate social support
– Inadequate knowledge of treatment regimen
– Ineffective coping skills
– Negative feelings toward treatment regimen
– Nonacceptance of condition
– Unrealistic perception of seriousness of condition
– Perceived social stigma associated with condition
– Unrealistic perception of treatment benefit

The nurse also collected the following data, which would be interpreted as defining characteristics for this diagnosis:

– Caregiver strain
– Depressive symptoms of caregiver
– Exacerbation of disease signs of one or more family members
– Exacerbation of disease symptoms of one or more family members
– Ineffective choices in daily living for meeting health goal of family unit
– One or more family members report dissatisfaction with quality of life

Although nurses cannot independently intervene upon at risk populations or associated conditions, it is important to be aware of individuals for whom a nursing diagnosis might be more likely to occur. Thus, the nurse should have identified the following at risk population that would potentially alert the nurse to concerns for this diagnosis:

– Economically disadvantaged families

Listed below are some examples of nursing goals, outcomes and actions, primarily linked to etiological factors. This is not presented as a comprehensive plan of care, but rather provides examples to demonstrate the proper method for linking diagnosis to outcomes and interventions, in an evidence-based manner.

Mr. F.F.J.'s family nursing diagnosis, ultimate goal, outcomes and nursing actions

Nursing diagnosis	Ineffective family health self-management (00294)	
Ultimate goal(s)	Effective family health self-management	
Related factors	Outcomes	Nursing actions
Competing demands on family unit	Prioritization of demands in the family unit	Assist with prioritization of demands
Conflict between spiritual beliefs and treatment regimen	Balance between spiritual beliefs and treatment regimen	Discuss spiritual beliefs, positive and negative aspects of the treatment, and evolution of the disease

Defining characteristics	Outcomes	Nursing actions
Difficulty dealing with role changes associated with condition	Coping with role changes associated with health condition	Assist caregiver in planning strategies for coping with role changes
Family conflict	Absence of family conflict	Promote active listening with caregiver and family members
Unsupportive family relations	Adequate family communication Supportive family relations	Assist with non-violent communication techniques
Inadequate social support	Adequate social support	Identify and provide information on support groups providing local or online support to individuals with chronic disease
Inadequate knowledge of treatment regimen	Adequate knowledge of treatment regimen	Educate the extended family on the treatment regimen benefits
Ineffective coping skills	Effective coping skills	Assist with coping techniques
Negative feelings toward treatment regimen	Positive feelings toward treatment regimen	Allow for the expression of negative feelings about the health condition and treatment
Nonacceptance of condition	Acceptance of condition	Explain and illustrate seriousness of condition
Unrealistic perception of seriousness of condition	Realistic perception of seriousness of condition	
Perceived social stigma associated with condition	Coping with the perceived social stigma associated with the health condition	Educate the family about stigmas associated with the health condition Educate the community about stigmas associated with the health condition
Unrealistic perception of treatment benefit	Realistic perception of treatment benefit	Clarify doubts about the treatment, duration and effectiveness
Defining characteristics	**Outcomes**	**Nursing actions**
Caregiver strain	Caregiver well-being	Monitor level of caregiver strain using standardized, validated tool
Depressive symptoms of caregiver	Improvement in depressive symptoms	Monitor severity of depressive symptoms using standardized, validated tool Let caregiver know her feelings matter

Exacerbation of disease signs of one or more family members	Absence of disease signs in family members Improvement in disease signs in family members	Educate on self-monitoring of disease symptoms Monitor severity of disease signs of one or more family members
Exacerbation of disease symptoms of one or more family members	Absence of disease signs in family members Improvement in disease signs in family members	Educate on self-monitoring of disease symptoms Monitor severity of disease signs in family members

Domain 1 • Class 2 • Diagnosis Code 00300

Ineffective home maintenance behaviors

T. Heather Herdman

NANDA International, Inc. Nursing Diagnoses: Definitions and Classification 2021–2023, 12th Edition, p. 206

Definition
An unsatisfactory pattern of knowledge and activities for the safe upkeep of one's residence, which may compromise health.

Model case

M.M. & J.M. are a couple in their late 20 s with a 3-year old daughter, S.M. During a visit to the pediatric clinic, S.M. was noted to have a skin rash that was linked to bed bugs. She had areas of raised red welts across her left flank and on her forearms and legs. She indicated that these areas itched, and sometimes they hurt. It was also noted that her clothes were dirty, and her hair didn't appear to have been washed recently. S.M.'s father, J.M., is known to have a history of significant clinical depression, and her mother, M.M., works two jobs to provide for the family.

A home visit was scheduled, and on arrival, the house is cluttered with empty beverage and take out food containers, dirty clothes are piled on the floor in both bedrooms, and the kitchen is full of dirty dishes that appear to represent several days of food preparation and consumption. The bathroom is dirty, mold is apparent in the shower, and towels are in a pile on the floor. M.M. comments that she is overwhelmed with the housework. "'I'm exhausted from working 12 hours a day for 6 days a week. I look at the house and I never know where to start, and I can't decide, and then I get stressed, and I can't function like that, so it just never gets done. Then the next day it's all worse, and J.M. and I fight about it all the time."

S.M.'s room has boxes all over the floor with what appear to be some clothes to be packed away, but the project seems to have been abandoned without being finished. It is impossible to walk within the room without having to step over a box. M.M. indicates that she can't decide what to put in which box, and she has so many tasks to complete that she can't seem to do any of them. There is nowhere to put the boxes once they're packed, due to a lack of storage space in the house, so she doesn't know what to do. She becomes agitated while talking about maintaining the household in a way to assure safety and cleanliness. J.M. remains completely unengaged during the entire visit.

Assessment

During the assessment, the nurse collected the following data, which could be interpreted to be related (causative) factors for this diagnosis:
- Depressive symptoms
- Difficulty with decision-making
- Environmental constraints
- Inadequate organizational skills
- Psychological distress

The nurse also collected the following data, which would be interpreted as defining characteristics for this diagnosis:
- Cluttered environment
- Difficulty maintaining a comfortable environment
- Home task-related anxiety
- Home task-related stress
- Neglected laundry
- Trash accumulation
- Unsanitary environment

Although nurses cannot independently intervene upon at risk populations or associated conditions, it is important to be aware of individuals for whom a nursing diagnosis might be more likely to occur. The assessment would have identified the following associated conditions that should alert the nurse to consider the possibility of this diagnosis:
- Depression
- Mental disorders

Listed below are some examples of nursing goals, outcomes and actions, primarily linked to etiological factors. This is not presented as a comprehensive plan of care, but rather provides examples to demonstrate the proper method for linking diagnosis to outcomes and interventions, in an evidence-based manner.

M.M & J.M.'s nursing diagnosis, ultimate goal, outcomes and nursing actions

Nursing diagnosis	Ineffective home maintenance behaviors (00300)	
Ultimate goal(s)	Effective home maintenance behaviors	
Related factor	**Outcome**	**Nursing actions**
Depressive symptoms Psychological distress	Depressive symptoms remain stable Improvement in depressive symptoms Stabilized mood	Focus discussion on feelings Demonstrate acceptance and understanding of the depressive symptoms. Use silence and active listening during interactions Monitor severity of depressive symptoms using a standardized, validated tool Refer to specialized psychological care, as needed
Difficulty with decision-making	Adequate decision-making skills Shared parental decision-making	Utilize shared decision-making to support family in improving skills

Environmental constraints	Environment is safe Environment is clean	Assess living space for safety and hygiene, using a standardized, validated assessment tool Educate parents on environmental safety to prevent illness and injury
Inadequate organizational skills	Adequate organizational skills	Assess ability to manage home maintenance independently
Inadequate knowledge of home maintenance	Adequate knowledge of home maintenance	Educate on home maintenance needs Teach home maintenance skills to maintain safety and hygiene
Inadequate knowledge of social resources	Adequate knowledge of social resources	Provide information on available social services and what services are provided Support in obtaining available resources

Domain 1 • Class 2 • Diagnosis Code 00308

Risk for ineffective home maintenance behaviors

T. Heather Herdman

NANDA International, Inc. Nursing Diagnoses: Definitions and Classification 2021–2023, 12th Edition, p. 207

Definition

Susceptible to an unsatisfactory pattern of knowledge and activities for the safe upkeep of one's residence, which may compromise health.

Model case

J.H. is a 25-year-old man with a history of severe malnourishment during the first seven years of his life, when he was housed in an orphanage. As a result, he has diminished intellectual performance, low work capacity, and an increased risk of immune-related conditions. He also has delayed motor abilities and finds some social situations awkward due to a lack of social skills and boundaries.

J.H. has been living with his adoptive parents, but now wishes to move into an apartment to have more independence. His parents support his move toward autonomy but worry about his ability to maintain a home setting that will be safe, clean, and prevent unnecessary exposure to pathogens. He has participated in home maintenance skills at his parents' home, but always with guidance, so they worry that he may not be able to manage on his own. His parents comment that they have perhaps not helped him develop good organizational skills himself because they always maintained a list of tasks for him to accomplish each day, rather than having him learn to organize his own needs over time.

J.H. also says he has some worries, mostly that he tires easily because of his mobility challenges and his congenital aortic valve stenosis. He worries this will keep him from being successful maintaining his living space on his own. He notes that he struggles with decision-making and becomes easily overwhelmed when there is more than one demand placed on him at a time.

Assessment

During the assessment, the nurse collected the following data, which could be interpreted to be risk (causative/predisposing) factors for this diagnosis:
- Cognitive dysfunction
- Competing demands
- Difficulty with decision-making
- Impaired physical mobility
- Inadequate knowledge of home maintenance
- Inadequate knowledge of social resources

Listed below are some examples of nursing goals, outcomes and actions, linked to etiological factors. This is not presented as a comprehensive plan of care, but rather provides examples to demonstrate the proper method for linking diagnosis to outcomes and interventions, in an evidence-based manner.

H.W.'s nursing diagnosis, ultimate goal, outcomes and nursing actions

Nursing diagnosis	Risk for ineffective home maintenance behaviors (00308)	
Ultimate goal(s)	Effective home maintenance behaviors	
Risk Factor	Outcome	Nursing actions
Cognitive dysfunction	Adequate organizational skills	Assess client's ability to manage home maintenance independently Consider referral for cognitive training Support in developing organizational checklists for home maintenance
Competing demands	Develops plan to prioritize demands	Support in developing methods to prioritize demands
Difficulty with decision-making	Adequate decision-making skills	Utilize shared decision-making to support client in improving his skill
Impaired physical mobility	Adequate physical mobility	Consider home repairs and modifications, as needed Assess living space for safety, using a standardized, validated assessment tool Educate client on home safety needs Teach and reinforce home safety skills Encourage physical activity to encourage balance and avert falls at least 3x/week
Inadequate knowledge of home maintenance	Adequate knowledge of home maintenance	Assess living space for safety and hygiene, using a standardized, validated assessment tool Educate client on home maintenance needs Teach home maintenance skills to maintain safety and hygiene
Inadequate knowledge of social resources	Adequate knowledge of social resources	Provide information on available social services and what services are provided Support in obtaining available resources

Domain 1 • Class 2 • Diagnosis Code 00309

Readiness for enhanced home maintenance behaviors

T. Heather Herdman

NANDA International, Inc. Nursing Diagnoses: Definitions and Classification 2021–2023, 12th Edition, p. 208

Definition
A pattern of knowledge and activities for the safe upkeep of one's residence, which can be strengthened.

Model case

M.M. & J.M. are a couple in their late 20 s with a 3-year old daughter, S.M. This family entered into care with the home health agency about six months ago, after the child was noted to have a skin rash that was linked to bed bugs. Her father, J.M., has a history of significant clinical depression, and her mother, M.M., works two jobs to provide for the family.

On the initial home visit, the house was cluttered and unsafe, dirty, and disorganized. S.M. verbalized feelings of being overwhelmed and exhausted due to working two jobs and trying to care for her husband, daughter, and the home.

Since the original visit, J.M. has been receiving nursing support and psychological care for his depression and has begun to participate in household activities. M.M. has been working with a social support group in her community to learn new coping strategies for stress, such as meditation. On this visit, the nurse sees that the kitchen is free from dirty dishes, and the house is clean, although still somewhat cluttered. However, there are clear pathways in each room, so the safety aspects are much better than on the first visit.

In talking about their progress, both of the parents indicated that they were proud of the work they have accomplished, and that they feel less stressed and more in control of their daily lives. J.M. indicates that they have been discussing their desire to enhance the safety and comfort of their home, and to improve their organizational skills, and he has begun to look for a part-time job to decrease the stress on M.M.

Assessment

During the assessment, the nurse collected the following data, which would be interpreted as defining characteristics of motivation and desire to increase well-being and to actualize health potential:

– Expresses desire to enhance comfort of the environment

– Expresses desire to enhance home safety
– Expresses desire to enhance organizational skills

Listed below are some examples of nursing goals, outcomes and actions. This is not presented as a comprehensive plan of care, but rather provides examples to demonstrate the proper method for linking diagnosis to outcomes and interventions, in an evidence-based manner.

M.M & J.M.'s nursing diagnosis, ultimate goal, outcomes and nursing actions

Nursing diagnosis	Readiness for enhanced home maintenance behaviors (00309)	
Ultimate goal(s)	Enhanced home maintenance behaviors	
Defining Characteristics	**Outcome**	**Nursing actions**
Expresses desire to enhance comfort of the environment	Enhanced comfort of the environment	Encourage to determine mid-range goals for home maintenance Provide support for organizing home to improve environmental comfort Identify and encourage outreach to neighborhood support organizations for improving environmental comfort
Expresses desire to enhance home safety	Enhanced home safety	Assess living space for safety and hygiene, using a standardized, validated assessment tool Reinforce home safety needs Reinforce home safety skills Provide positive feedback on achievements Identify and encourage outreach to neighborhood support organizations for improving environmental safety
Expresses desire to enhance organizational skills	Enhanced organizational skills	Reinforce skills for organizing the environment Reinforce use of checklists for organization of home maintenance tasks Provide positive feedback on achievements Identify and encourage outreach to neighborhood support organizations for improving organizational skills

Domain 2.
Nutrition

Class 1.   Ingestion

Class 4.   Metabolism

Domain 2 • Class 1 • Diagnosis Code 00295

Ineffective infant suck-swallow response

T. Heather Herdman

NANDA International, Inc. Nursing Diagnoses: Definitions and Classification 2021–2023, 12th Edition, p. 232

Definition
Impaired ability of an infant to suck or to coordinate the suck-swallow response.

Model case
Infant T.B. is a 29-week gestation infant in the newborn step-down unit, where he is struggling to gain weight and maintain a normal body temperature. He is on an every three hour feeding schedule of maternal milk, but he struggles to bottle feed. During feedings, he exhibits multiple stress responses, including finger splaying, hiccups, and circumoral cyanosis. If bottle feedings persist, he becomes unable to coordinate sucking, swallowing and breathing, begins choking, and his overall muscle tone becomes flaccid. Finally, he begins to have subcostal retractions and/or uses accessory muscles to breathe, exhibits multiple time-out signals, and may experience several episodes of bradycardia, and/or oxygen desaturation.

He has more difficulty when his parents attempt to feed him, as they seem to be uncomfortable with positioning him appropriately. His father has said, "I'm just afraid I'm going to break him, he's so fragile".

Assessment
During the assessment, the nurse collected the following data, which could be interpreted to be related (causative) factors for this diagnosis:
- Hypothermia
- Inappropriate positioning
- Unsatisfactory sucking behavior

The nurse also collected the following data, which would be interpreted as defining characteristics for this diagnosis:
- Bradycardic events
- Choking
- Circumoral cyanosis
- Excessive coughing
- Finger splaying
- Flaccidity
- Hiccups
- Impaired motor tone

- Inability to coordinate sucking, swallowing, and breathing
- Oxygen desaturation
- Subcostal retraction
- Time-out signals
- Uses accessory muscles to breathe

Although nurses cannot independently intervene upon at risk populations or associated conditions, it is important to be aware of individuals for whom a nursing diagnosis might be more likely to occur. Thus, the nurse should have identified the following at risk population that would potentially alert the nurse to concerns for this diagnosis:

- Premature infants

Listed below are some examples of nursing goals, outcomes and actions, primarily linked to etiological factors. This is not presented as a comprehensive plan of care, but rather provides examples to demonstrate the proper method for linking diagnosis to outcomes and interventions, in an evidence-based manner.

T.B.'s nursing diagnosis, ultimate goal, outcomes and nursing actions

Nursing diagnosis	Ineffective infant suck-swallow response (00295)	
Ultimate goal(s)	Effective infant suck-swallow response	
Related factors	**Outcomes**	**Nursing actions**
Hypothermia	Normothermia	Initiate skin-to-skin contact with parent(s) as possible Maintain infant in climate controlled isolette/warming table, when not on parent's chest Educate parents on methods to manage thermoregulation in newborn Ensure parents can verbalize methods to promote and maintain normothermia in infant
Inappropriate positioning	Appropriate infant positioning	Guide parents in therapeutic positioning of infant for feeding Encourage use of semi-elevated side-lying position during infant feeding
Unsatisfactory sucking behavior	Satisfactory sucking behavior	Use standardized, validated tool to assess infant readiness for and tolerance of feeding and to profile infant's developmental stage regarding specific feeding skills Conserve energy by decreasing stimuli to infant, as possible Teach caregiver to observe infant cues of stress during feeding Allow for rest periods for reorganization of infant swallowing function Offer opportunities for deep breathing and brief resting periods while feeding Consider supplementing feedings using oral gastric tube until stable

2. Nutrition

Domain 2 • Class 4 • Diagnosis Code 00241

Risk for metabolic syndrome

T. Heather Herdman

NANDA International, Inc. Nursing Diagnoses: Definitions and Classification 2021–2023, 12th Edition, p. 241

> **Definition**
> Susceptible to developing a cluster of symptoms that increase risk of cardio-vascular disease and type 2 diabetes mellitus, which may compromise health.

Model case

Ms. J.T. is an obese 32-year old teacher, who smokes and admits to drinking 3–4 alcoholic beverages a night, with more on the weekend. She states, "I'm young and I like to party, what's wrong with that?" She states that after she comes home, she either meets a friend at a fast food restaurant for dinner, or she heats a frozen meal in the microwave. She will then have 2–3 glasses of wine while she watches TV until bedtime. She gets up in the morning, goes through a drive to a coffee shop for a sweetened coffee beverage and a bakery item, and then eats from the cafeteria for lunch.

Her parents and her one sibling are overweight or obese, and her father has type 2 diabetes. She denies any concern regarding her health and indicates no interest in changing her behaviors. J.T. says, "Why shouldn't I eat what I want? You only live once."

Assessment

During the assessment, the nurse collected the following data, which could be interpreted to be risk (causative/predisposing) factors for this diagnosis:
- Absence of interest in improving health behaviors
- Average daily physical activity is less than recommended for age and gender
- Body mass index above normal range for age and gender
- Excessive accumulation of fat for age and gender
- Excessive alcohol consumption
- Inadequate dietary habits
- Smoking

Although nurses cannot independently intervene upon at risk populations or associated conditions, it is important to be aware of individuals for whom a nursing diagnosis might be more likely to occur. Thus, the nurse should have identified the following at risk populations that would potentially alert the nurse to concerns for this diagnosis:
- Individuals aged > 30 years

–   Individuals with family history of diabetes mellitus
–   Individuals with family history of obesity

Listed below are some examples of nursing goals, outcomes and actions, linked to etiological factors. This is not presented as a comprehensive plan of care, but rather provides examples to demonstrate the proper method for linking diagnosis to outcomes and interventions, in an evidence-based manner.

J.T.'s nursing diagnosis, ultimate goal, outcomes and nursing actions

Nursing diagnosis	Risk for metabolic syndrome (00241)	
Ultimate goal(s)	Prevention of metabolic syndrome	
Risk factors	**Outcomes**	**Nursing actions**
Absence of interest in improving health behaviors	Desire to improve health behaviors	Establish and maintain trust building between client and nurse Provide stability and consistency in nursing caregivers to enable relationship building and establish trust Provide a non-judgmental approach Provide in-home, nurse-delivered and culturally sensitive education and home visit intervention targeting metabolic syndrome prevention Educate on risk factors Identify and provide information on support groups providing local or online support to individuals with risk for metabolic syndrome
Average daily physical activity is less than recommended for age and gender	Engages in recommended average daily physical activity	Support client in goal-setting Provide adherence counseling Assist in identifying peer support group / community center who might support client in adopting new physical activities
Inadequate dietary habits Body mass index above normal range for age and gender Excessive accumulation of fat for age and gender	Adequate dietary habits Body mass index normal range for age and gender Fat stores average for age and gender	Support client in determining short-, medium-, and long-term goals for weight reduction Establish a realistic plan for weight loss, with client, by reducing foods that are high in saturated fats and carbohydrates, replacing them with healthier food, and increasing energy expenditure Consider use of social media and online applications to support lifestyle changes Identify and provide information on support groups for individuals wanting to improve dietary habits Support client in determining short-, medium-, and long-term goals for physical activity

2. Nutrition

Excessive alcohol consumption	Normal alcohol consumption	Provide education on linkages between depression and alcohol consumption
Smoking	Smoking cessation	Offer smoking cessation counseling
		Refer for motivational interviewing or cognitive behavior therapy focused on smoking cessation and alcohol reduction
		Refer to pharmacotherapy program for smoking cessation if needed
		Consider cognitive behavioral therapy for alcohol reduction
		Identify and provide information on support groups for individuals wanting to undertake lifestyle changes
		Encourage sharing of feelings and concerns

Domain 3.
Elimination and exchange

Class 1.   Urinary function

Code	Diagnosis	Page
00297	Disability-associated urinary incontinence	72
00310	Mixed urinary incontinence	74
00322	Risk for urinary retention	77

Class 2.   Gastrointestinal function

Code	Diagnosis	Page
00319	Impaired bowel continence	79

Domain 3 • Class 1 • Diagnosis Code 00297

Disability-associated urinary incontinence

Camila Takáo Lopes, Juliana Neves da Costa

NANDA International, Inc. Nursing Diagnoses: Definitions and Classification 2021–2023, 12th Edition, p. 249

Definition
Involuntary loss of urine not associated with any pathology or problem related to the urinary system.

Model case
J.P., a 5-year-old girl, had her right ankle broken two weeks ago and is currently wearing a cask and needs crutches to walk. She loves her art classes at school. When picking J.P. up from school in the past two weeks, her mother, Mrs. B.T.P., was informed by J.P.'s teacher that she had urinated in her pants. She tells Mrs. B.T.P. that J.P. kept crossing her legs, and moving back and forth restlessly during class. When she finally decided to tell the teacher that she needed to rush to the bathroom, she urinated before they could get to the bathroom. J.P. says that she is postponing going to the bathroom because she is afraid to miss out on the art activities. Mrs. B.T.P. also noticed that this sometimes occurs when J.P. is rushing to the bathroom to urinate at home, when she is watching her favorite show on TV.

Assessment
During the assessment, the nurse collected the following data, which could be interpreted to be related (causative) factors for this diagnosis:
–   Habitually suppresses urge to urinate
The nurse would also have collected the following data, which would be interpreted as defining characteristics for this diagnosis:
–   Use of techniques to prevent urination
–   Voiding prior to reaching toilet
Although nurses cannot independently intervene upon at risk populations or associated conditions, it is important to be aware of individuals for whom a nursing diagnosis might be more likely to occur. Thus, the nurse should have identified the following at risk population that would potentially alert the nurse to concerns for this diagnosis:
–   Children
Listed below are some examples of nursing goals, outcomes and actions, primarily linked to etiological factors. This is not presented as a comprehensive plan of care, but rather provides examples to demonstrate the proper method for linking diagnosis to outcomes and interventions, in an evidence-based manner.

J.P.'s family nursing diagnosis, ultimate goal, outcomes and nursing actions

Nursing diagnosis	Disability-associated urinary incontinence (00297)	
Ultimate goal(s)	Urinary continence	
Related factors	**Outcomes**	**Nursing actions**
Habitually suppresses urge to urinate	Habitually meets urge to urinate	Educate teacher and parents on timed voiding schedule, aimed at five to seven voids per day, in regular intervals of 1½–3 h Educate teacher and parents on using reminders (e.g., digital wrist alarm watches with auditory or vibratory signals, count-down timers or smart phones set to remind the child to go to the toilet) Educate teacher, parents, and child to note micturition in the toilet and wetting episodes in a chart Educate child to sit on the toilet in a relaxed way and take plenty of time Educate teacher and parents to use positive reinforcement
Defining characteristics	**Outcomes**	**Nursing actions**
Use of techniques to prevent urination	Does not prevent urination	Monitor for use of techniques to prevent urination Encourage child to self-monitor for the use of techniques to prevent urination
Voiding prior to reaching toilet	Voiding when reaching toilet	Monitor for voiding management by the child Refer to specialist to rule out neurogenic and other organic causes if voiding prior to reaching toilet persists

Domain 3 • Class 1 • Diagnosis Code 00310

Mixed urinary incontinence

Juliana Neves da Costa, Camila Takáo Lopes

NANDA International, Inc. Nursing Diagnoses: Definitions and Classification 2021–2023, 12th Edition, p. 251

Definition
Involuntary loss of urine in combination with or following a strong sensation or urgency to void, and also with activities that increase intra-abdominal pressure.

Model case
Mrs. T.R. is a mother of four who gave birth vaginally. Eight months following her last delivery, she started noticing that she urinated while coughing and sneezing. She also frequently has a sudden, uncontrollable need to urinate and has to rush to the bathroom. She has not managed to lose the weight she gained during pregnancy, and her hectic routine with the children has made it impossible to practice regular physical exercise. She refers to a sensation of a lump in her vagina, especially when she spends long periods of time standing. She feels that her vagina is "loose" and that it is difficult for her to contract her pelvic floor muscles during sexual intercourse or when she is trying to prevent urinary leakage. She indicates that she is not a smoker, and has two bowel movements daily.

Assessment
During the assessment, the nurse collected the following data, which could be interpreted to be related (causative) factors for this diagnosis:
– Overweight
– Pelvic floor disorders
– Pelvic organ prolapse
– Skeletal muscular atrophy
The nurse also collected the following data, which would be interpreted as defining characteristics for this diagnosis:
– Involuntary loss of urine upon coughing
– Involuntary loss of urine upon sneezing
– Urinary urgency
Although nurses cannot intervene upon populations who are at risk for a condition, or associated conditions, it is important to be aware of individuals for whom a nursing diagnosis might be more likely to occur. Thus, the nurse should have identified the following at risk populations that would potentially alert the nurse to concerns for this diagnosis:

- Multiparous women
- Women giving birth vaginally

Listed below are some examples of nursing goals, outcomes and actions, primarily linked to etiological factors. This is not presented as a comprehensive plan of care, but rather provides examples to demonstrate the proper method for linking diagnosis to outcomes and interventions, in an evidence-based manner.

T.R.'s family nursing diagnosis, ultimate goal, outcomes and nursing actions

Nursing diagnosis	Mixed urinary incontinence (00310)	
Ultimate goal(s)	Urinary continence	
Related factors	**Outcomes**	**Nursing actions**
Overweight	Normal weight for height, weight, and gender	Assist with prioritizing competing demands Assist in identifying peer support group that might assist with food preparation and/or exercise routine Establish a realistic plan for weight loss, with client, by reducing foods that are high in saturated fats and carbohydrates, replacing them with healthier food, and increasing energy expenditure Encourage regular exercise for about 150 minutes a week
Skeletal muscular atrophy	Strengthened pelvic muscles	Educate to identify pelvic floor muscles Educate to isolate accessory muscles during contraction and relaxation of pelvic floor muscles Establish an individualized pelvic floor muscle strengthening program, providing education on strengthening and relaxation of these muscles Teach to contract and relax muscle around the urethra and anus Refer to pelvic floor rehabilitation specialist if there is no improvement in 4 weeks
Pelvic floor disorders	Improved functioning of pelvic muscles	
Pelvic organ prolapse	Reduced pelvic organ prolapse	Recommend vaginal pessary and discuss follow-up regimen with client Educate on insertion and retention of vaginal pessary Educate to identify and manage the most common complications of vatinal pessary use

3. Elimination and exchange

3. Elimination and exchange

Defining characteristics	Outcomes	Nursing actions
Involuntary loss of urine upon coughing	Urine continence when coughing	Educate on incorporating the "knack" maneuver into daily living
Involuntary loss of urine upon sneezing	Urine continence when sneezing	
Urinary urgency	Decreased urinary urgency	Educate on use of a diary for self-monitoring of urinary elimination, including frequency, interval between urinations, volume, episodes of urgency and urinary loss, type and amount of fluids ingested Identify factors that contribute to episodes of urgency and incontinence Educate on controlling factors identified that may contribute to episodes of urgency and incontinence Educate on bladder training techniques

Domain 3 • Class 1 • Diagnosis Code 00322

Risk for urinary retention

Meiry Fernanda Pinto Okuno, Camila Takáo Lopes

NANDA International, Inc. Nursing Diagnoses: Definitions and Classification 2021–2023, 12th Edition, p. 256

Definition
Susceptible to incomplete emptying of the bladder.

Model case
Nurse Denise is conducting a home visit to Mrs. A.F.P., for the Multidimensional Assessment of the Elderly. Mrs. A.F.P. is a 75-year-old retired secretary, mother of three, living with her 80-year-old husband, who is bedridden. She reports pelvic pain and discomfort due to uterine prolapse and weakened bladder muscles as a result of two natural deliveries and one forceps delivery; she also reports taking care of her husband alone, so she is always busy and holding her urine for a long time. When she finally goes to the restroom, she adopts a near-standing posture to urinate.

Assessment
During the assessment, the nurse collected the following data, which could be interpreted to be risk (causative/predisposing) factors for this diagnosis:
–   Improper toileting posture
–   Pelvic organ prolapse
–   Weakened bladder muscle
Listed below are some examples of nursing goals, outcomes and actions, linked to etiological factors. This is not presented as a comprehensive plan of care, but rather provides examples to demonstrate the proper method for linking diagnosis to outcomes and interventions, in an evidence-based manner.

A.F.P.'s nursing diagnosis, ultimate goal, outcomes and nursing actions

Nursing diagnosis	Risk for urinary retention (00322)	
Ultimate goal(s)	Complete bladder emptying	
Risk factors	**Outcomes**	**Nursing actions**
Improper toileting posture	Proper toileting posture	Assist with planning of care activities Educate on timed voids and not holding urine Educate to always sit down on toilet with feet supported and to relax pelvic muscles
Pelvic organ prolapse	Maintenance of current level of pelvic organ prolapse	Recommend vaginal pessary and discuss follow-up regimen with client Educate on insertion and retention of vaginal pessary Educate to identify and manage the most common complications of vaginal pessary use
Weakened bladder muscle	Strengthened bladder muscle	Educate on pelvic floor strengthening exercises

Domain 3 • Class 2 • Diagnosis Code 00319

Impaired bowel continence

T. Heather Herdman

NANDA International, Inc. Nursing Diagnoses: Definitions and Classification 2021–2023, 12th Edition, p. 265

> **Definition**
> Inability to hold stool, to sense the presence of stool in the rectum, to relax and store stool when having a bowel movement is not convenient.

Model case

Mrs. T.S. is a 89-year-old woman who reports overall good health, but has come to the clinic due to concerns of bowel incontinence. She takes arthritis and pain medications, says she eats two meals a day, and generally feels good except for significant arthritis in her hips, knees, hands and neck.

However, in the past few months she has started to have difficulty with her bowels, and has noticed staining of her undergarments upon awakening, which has now increased to 3–4 times per week. She has also started to have bowel incontinence episodes during the day in the past two months, as often as 2–3 times per week, predominantly while taking a walk or going to the grocery store, where the bathroom is a long distance from many aisles in the store. She does indicate that she moves very slowly due to her arthritis and her age, and she states she is weaker than when she was younger. She reports that she needs to continue to walk as much as she can, as this helps with the pain in her joints.

Mrs. T.S. lives alone and says that she will suddenly realize she needs to have a bowel movement, but cannot get to the bathroom in time, nor can she prevent herself from defecating. She is now wearing incontinence briefs, but she is very unhappy with this situation.

Assessment

During the assessment, the nurse collected the following data, which could be interpreted to be related (causative) factors for this diagnosis:
- Generalized decline in muscle tone
- Impaired physical mobility
- Environmental constraints that interfere with continence

The nurse also collected the following data, which would be interpreted as defining characteristics for this diagnosis:
- Bowel urgency
- Fecal staining
- Inability to delay defecation

- Inability to reach toilet in time
- Silent leakage of stool during activities

Although nurses cannot independently intervene upon at risk populations or associated conditions, it is important to be aware of individuals for whom a nursing diagnosis might be more likely to occur. Thus, the nurse should have identified the following at risk population that would potentially alert the nurse to concerns for this diagnosis:

- Older adults

Listed below are some examples of nursing goals, outcomes and actions, primarily linked to etiological factors. This is not presented as a comprehensive plan of care, but rather provides examples to demonstrate the proper method for linking diagnosis to outcomes and interventions, in an evidence-based manner.

T.S.'s nursing diagnosis, ultimate goal, outcomes and nursing actions

Nursing diagnosis	Impaired bowel continence (00319)	
Ultimate goal(s)	Bowel continence	
Related factors	**Outcomes**	**Nursing actions**
Generalized decline in muscle tone	Improved muscle tone	Educate on pelvic floor exercises to strengthen area of anus and rectum
		Consider pelvic floor biofeedback therapy
		Teach and monitor progress with stretching exercises
		Teach and monitor progress with muscle strengthening and resistance exercises at least 2x/week
		Begin with lower-intensity activities and progressively advance onto moderate or higher-impact activities, working toward 150 minutes or aerobic physical activity consistently each week
		Consider Vitamin D therapy 700 IU/d to 1000 IU/d for improved muscle strength and balance
Impaired physical mobility	Improved physical mobility	Assess living space for safety, using a standardized, validated assessment tool
		Educate client on home safety needs
		Teach and reinforce home safety skills
		Teach and monitor progress with bone strengthening exercises
		Encourage physical activity to encourage balance and avert falls at least 3x/week

Environmental constraints that interfere with continence	Improved bowel continence	Educate to refrain from ingesting caffeine, citrus fruits, spicy foods, and alcohol, which have the effect of softening the stool
		Educate to include dietary fiber, such as psyllium, in daily diet
		Initiate defecation habit training twice a day (approximately 30 minutes after breakfast or dinner)
		Encourage activity that places client far from restroom immediately after defecation
		Refer to bowel continence program, if available

3. Elimination and exchange

Domain 4.
Activity/rest

Class 2. Activity/exercise

Code	Diagnosis	Page
00298	Decreased activity tolerance	84
00299	Risk for decreased activity tolerance	86

Class 4. Cardiovascular/pulmonary responses

Code	Diagnosis	Page
00311	Risk for impaired cardiovascular function	88
00278	Ineffective lymphedema self-management	90
00281	Risk for ineffective lymphedema self-management	94
00291	Risk for thrombosis	97
00318	Dysfunctional adult ventilatory weaning response	99

Domain 4 • Class 2 • Diagnosis Code 00298

Decreased activity tolerance

Camila Takáo Lopes, Beatriz Murata Murakami

NANDA International, Inc. Nursing Diagnoses: Definitions and Classification 2021–2023, 12th Edition, p. 280

Definition
Insufficient endurance to complete required or desired daily activities.

Model case
Mrs. S.H., 52 years old, sprained her right ankle 30 days ago after slipping on the bathroom floor. She was diagnosed with a minor sprain and instructed to rest and avoid activities that could cause pain or worsen the edema, to use ice packs 4 to 8 times a day for 15 minutes, to compress her ankle with an elastic bandage, and to keep her right lower limb elevated for 15 days. She was provided with crutches to help her walk and over-the-counter pain relievers were prescribed. She slept on the couch downstairs and followed instructions for 15 days, but she refused to walk with or without the aid of crutches because she was too afraid of worsening the pain and of falling again. Instead, her daughter has been helping her around the house with a borrowed wheelchair.

The edema is much better, and her level of pain decreased from an 8 to a 3 out of 10, so she was told to begin exercises to restore her ankle's range of motion, strength, flexibility, and stability. She has been trying to perform her usual daily living activities and to exercise for the past 15 days, but she feels uncomfortable and has to sit down, so whenever she thinks of getting up and walking around, she gets really anxious. She is also afraid that her pain intensity will increase to an 8 again. In the past week, she has become apathetic and says that she does not feel well rested, even when she sleeps for eight hours.

Assessment
During the assessment, the nurse collected the following data, which could be interpreted to be related (causative) factors for this diagnosis:
- Fear of pain
- Impaired physical mobility
- Pain

The nurse also collected the following data, which would be interpreted as defining characteristics for this diagnosis:
- Anxious when activity is required
- Exertional discomfort
- Expresses fatigue

Listed below are some examples of nursing goals, outcomes and actions, primarily linked to etiological factors. This is not presented as a comprehensive plan of care, but rather provides examples to demonstrate the proper method for linking diagnosis to outcomes and interventions, in an evidence-based manner.

S.H.'s nursing diagnosis, ultimate goal, outcomes and nursing actions

Nursing diagnosis	Decreased activity tolerance (00298)	
Ultimate goal(s)	Activity tolerance	
Related factors	**Outcomes**	**Nursing actions**
Fear of pain	Improved fear of pain	Educate on misconceptions about the recovery and rehabilitation periods
Pain	Improved pain Absence of pain	Optimize prescribed medication for pain Educate caregiver to maintain observation during exercise, and reassure client Reach agreement on gradual increase of activities with and without assistance Plan for rest periods Educate on use of ice pack and rest if pain is present after walking
Impaired physical mobility	Adequate physical mobility	Educate client and caregiver on performing prescribed exercises slowly Monitor and correct exercises as needed Educate client and caregiver on performing activities of daily living slowly Reach agreement on rest periods according to level of energy Assist in prioritizing essential activities Teach energy conservation techniques
Defining characteristics	**Outcomes**	**Nursing actions**
Anxious when activity is required	Confident when activity is required	Monitor level of anxiety when activity is required Educate on misconceptions about the recovery and rehabilitation periods following ankle spraining Educate caregiver to maintain observation during exercise and reassure client
Exertional discomfort	Exertional comfort	Educate on self-monitoring of own limits Monitor level of exertional discomfort Monitor physiologic response to activity Encourage rest periods
Expresses fatigue	Expresses comfort	Educate on self-monitoring of own limits Monitor level of fatigue Encourage rest periods

4. Activity/rest

Domain 4 • Class 2 • Diagnosis Code 00299

Risk for decreased activity tolerance

Camila Takáo Lopes, Beatriz Murata Murakami

NANDA International, Inc. Nursing Diagnoses: Definitions and Classification 2021–2023, 12th Edition, p. 281

Definition
Susceptible to experiencing insufficient endurance to complete required or desired daily activities.

Model case
Mr. K.W., 52 years old, was diagnosed with heart failure with preserved ejection fraction six months ago, and was admitted to the hospital for acute decompensated heart failure five days ago. He had a complaint of worsening dyspnea on exertion, exertional fatigue, orthopnea, and paroxysmal nocturnal dyspnea. Upon physical examination, he had bibasilar crackles and lower limb edema bilaterally. During hospitalization, the nurse has been educated him and his son on health self-management focused on heart failure. After achieving clinical stability, he was discharged home.

Mr. K.W. tells the nurse that he has been feeling tearful, with a lack of energy, and has no motivation or interest in things. He finds it difficult to fall asleep and he wakes up very early in the morning, even when his heart failure is compensated, and he is not short of breath. Although he has a prescription for an exercise program and he is capable of performing activities of daily living without help, he has not engaged in exercise ever since he was a teenager. He believes his heart is weak, and exercising would put more stress on his heart.

Assessment
During the assessment, the nurse collected the following data, which could be interpreted to be risk (causative/predisposing) factors for this diagnosis:
- Depressive symptoms
- Sedentary lifestyle
- Inexperience with an activity

Listed below are some examples of nursing goals, outcomes and actions, linked to etiological factors. This is not presented as a comprehensive plan of care, but rather provides examples to demonstrate the proper method for linking diagnosis to outcomes and interventions, in an evidence-based manner.

K.W.'s nursing diagnosis, ultimate goal, outcomes and nursing actions

Nursing diagnosis	Risk for decreased activity tolerance (00299)	
Ultimate goal(s)	Activity tolerance	
Risk factors	**Outcomes**	**Nursing actions**
Depressive symptoms	Improvement in depressive symptoms	Monitor severity of depressive symptoms using a standardized, validated tool Focus discussion on feelings Demonstrate acceptance and understanding of the depressive symptoms Provide a non-judgmental approach Use silence and active listening during interactions Let client know that you are concerned and that his feelings matter Refer to specialized psychological care, as needed
Sedentary lifestyle Inexperience with activity	Active lifestyle Experience with activity	Educate on misconceptions about the rehabilitation period Encourage to determine gradual goals according to tolerance, starting with a reasonable short-term, medium-term, and long-term goal Encourage performance of light to moderate exercise for 30 minutes or more on most days of the week Educate to break exercise into intervals of 5 to 10 minutes across the day, if needed Encourage to use factual data chosen by the client to accompany exercise Educate on self-monitoring of ability to speak in full sentences and maintain a conversation comfortably during activity Encourage to progress exercise when current exercise program feels easy or light Educate on self-monitoring of progress in physical conditioning and physical well-being Educate on self-monitoring of signs of intolerance Incorporate regular supervision, feedback, and reinforcement strategies

4. Activity/rest

87

Domain 4 • Class 4 • Diagnosis Code 00311

Risk for impaired cardiovascular function

Juliana de Lima Lopes, Camila Takáo Lopes

NANDA International, Inc. Nursing Diagnoses: Definitions and Classification 2021–2023, 12ᵗʰ Edition, p. 300

Definition
Susceptible to disturbance in substance transport, body homeostasis, tissue metabolic residue removal, and organ function, which may compromise health.

Model case
Mrs. J.P.W., 41 years old, a single mother of two, has just been hired by a company as an executive secretary and is being assessed by the occupational health nurse. Mrs. J.P.W. had been under a lot of pressure in her previous job and had a hard time coping with her previous company's bankruptcy and dealing with six months of unemployment. She has been sitting at her computer from 8 a.m. to 6 p.m. daily, taking online courses and applying for new jobs. After 6 p.m., she picks up her 10-year-old child from school activities, so she has not been doing any physical activity.

She reports being a smoker for 20 years, and she currently smokes 2 packs of cigarettes per day. Her body mass index is currently 26 Kg/m² and her average blood pressure is 148 / 72 mmHg. When the nurse asks about her usual blood pressure, she says she never has it measured because she hardly ever adds salt to her food, but she has been eating a lot of deep-fried food lately. She reports that her mother has arterial hypertension and dyslipidemia, and her father experienced sudden death 10 years ago.

Assessment
During the assessment, the nurse collected the following data, which could be interpreted to be risk (causative/predisposing) factors for this diagnosis:
- Average daily physical activity is less than recommended for age and gender
- Excessive stress
- Inadequate knowledge of modifiable factors
- Ineffective blood pressure management
- Smoking

Although nurses cannot independently intervene upon at risk populations or associated conditions, it is important to be aware of individuals for whom a nursing diagnosis might be more likely to occur. Thus, the nurse should have

identified the following at risk population that would potentially alert the nurse to concerns for this diagnosis:
- Individuals with family history of hypertension

Listed below are some examples of nursing goals, outcomes and actions, linked to etiological factors. This is not presented as a comprehensive plan of care, but rather provides examples to demonstrate the proper method for linking diagnosis to outcomes and interventions, in an evidence-based manner.

J.P.W.'s nursing diagnosis, ultimate goal, outcomes and nursing actions

Nursing diagnosis	Risk for impaired cardiovascular function (00311)	
Ultimate goal(s)	Adequate cardiovascular function	
Risk factors	**Outcomes**	**Nursing actions**
Inadequate knowledge of modifiable factors	Adequate knowledge of modifiable factors	Educate on modifiable factors that increase cardiovascular risk
Average daily physical activity is less than recommended for age and gender	Average daily physical activity meets recommendations for age and gender	Assist with plan to increase physical activity according to tolerance and preferences Propose inclusion of family in physical activity
Excessive stress	Effective stress management	Educate on strategies for stress relief
Ineffective blood pressure management	Effective blood pressure management	Educate on regular blood pressure monitoring Educate to use blood pressure readings to support decision making
Smoking	Smoking cessation	Determine state of readiness for smoking reduction (pre-contemplation, contemplation, preparation) Refer for motivational interviewing or cognitive behavior therapy focused on smoking cessation Refer to pharmacotherapy program for smoking cessation, if needed Offer smoking cessation counseling Identify and provide information on support groups for individuals wanting to undertake lifestyle changes Consider use of social media and online applications to support lifestyle changes

Domain 4 • Class 4 • Diagnosis Code 00278

Ineffective lymphedema self-management

Edvane Birelo Lopes De Domenico, Camila Takáo Lopes

NANDA International, Inc. Nursing Diagnoses: Definitions and Classification 2021–2023, 12th Edition, p. 301

Definition
Unsatisfactory management of symptoms, treatment regimen, physical, psychosocial, and spiritual consequences and lifestyle changes inherent in living with edema related to obstruction or disorders of lymph vessels or nodes.

Model case
Mrs. J.Y. is a 65-year-old woman diagnosed with stage IV metastatic breast cancer (T4bN3M2) two years ago. Upon physical examination, a nodule can be found in her left breast, axillary, supraclavicular, and cervical lymph nodes. The histopathological result was an invasive ductal carcinoma grade 2; a luminal immunohistochemistry B, Ki67 20% (a protein in the breast cancer cell nucleus which is measured in % and reflects the rate of cell multiplication). Complementary exams showed multiple pulmonary nodular lesions, multiple bone metastases in the thoracic spine, sternum, ribs, and liver nodule. The proposed clinical treatment was intravenous antineoplastic chemotherapy associated with radiotherapy in the left breast and axillary regions, without a surgical indication. During the period of 25 radiotherapy sessions, the client was educated about the risks of lymphedema in the corresponding upper limb and the preventive measures that should be adopted. She had difficulty understanding the concept of lymphedema and the risk situation itself. She verbalized more than once that she didn't believe this could happen with radiotherapy alone and kept asking why she didn't have surgery.

After 6 months, Mrs. J.Y. started complaining of swelling, redness, tightness, and warmth of the skin on her left upper limb, characterizing a diagnosis of grade III neoplastic lymphedema, with restricted range of motion of the limb, monoplegia, pain and paresthesia. When asked about her daily activities, she reported performing all household activities, without any special attention to her left upper limb.

The proposed treatment plan for breast cancer-related lymphedema (BCRL) consisted of using a compression sleeve, education to perform passive exercises at home (elbow and hand) because of monoplegia, joint restriction of the affected shoulder, and a potent analgesic drug. In a face-to-face appointment with the nurse, the client reported not being able to perform the exercises due to constant pain. She has been avoiding using her compression sleeve because of the pain and because it keeps rolling down her arm. She has also been neglecting her treatment plan, such as not carrying weight using her left arm, because she was responsible for taking care of her 8-month-old granddaughter while her daughter worked. She stated that she does not know how she would be able to carry out the treatment for lymphedema, with the responsibility of helping her daughter and no one else to help her at home.

Assessment

During the assessment, the nurse collected the following data, which could be interpreted to be related (causative) factors for this diagnosis:
  – Competing demands
  – Inadequate social support
  – Limited ability to perform aspects of treatment regimen
The nurse also collected the following data, which would be interpreted as defining characteristics for this diagnosis:
      Lymphedema signs
  – Swelling in affected limb
Lymphedema symptoms
  – Reports feeling of discomfort in affected limb
  – Reports feeling of heaviness in affected limb
Behaviors
  – Inappropriate use of compression garments
  – Inattentive to carrying heavy objects
  – Reduced range of motion of affected limb
Although nurses cannot intervene upon populations who are at risk for a condition, it is important to be aware of individuals for whom a nursing diagnosis might be more likely to occur. Thus, the nurse should have identified the following at risk population and associated conditions that would potentially alert the nurse to concerns for this diagnosis:
  – Older adults
  – Individuals with history of Ineffective health self-management
  – Chemotherapy
  – Neoplasms
  – Radiotherapy
Listed below are some examples of nursing goals, outcomes and actions, primarily linked to etiological factors. This is not presented as a comprehensive plan of care, but rather provides examples to demonstrate the proper method for linking diagnosis to outcomes and interventions, in an evidence-based manner.

4. Activity/rest

4. Activity/rest

J.Y.'s nursing diagnosis, ultimate goal, outcomes and nursing actions

Nursing diagnosis	Ineffective lymphedema self-management (00278)	
Ultimate goal(s)	Effective lymphedema self-management	
Related factors	**Outcomes**	**Nursing actions**
Competing demands	Prioritization of competing demands	Assist with prioritizing competing demands
Inadequate social support	Adequate social support	Identify and provide information on support groups providing local or online support to individuals with chronic disease
		Assist in identifying peer support group who might assist with self-care or granddaughter's care
Limited ability to perform aspects of treatment regimen	Ability to perform treatment regimen	Discuss optimization of pain management for breast cancer-related lymphedema with provider
		Offer complementary/integrative health care options for pain relief, according to belief/preference
		Monitor for ability to perform exercises, initially supervised to ensure proper technique and progression
		Educate to avoid weight fluctuations during and after treatment
		Encourage maintenance of motor activity of the affected limb
		Reinforce importance of adherence to appointments for compression bandaging of the affected limb
		Monitor for and educate on self-monitoring of signs of infection, vascular congestion, sensory and motor changes in hand phalanges with compression bandaging
Defining characteristics	**Outcomes**	**Nursing actions**
Swelling in affected limb	Decreased swelling in affected limb	Educate on self-monitoring of swelling in affected limb
		Monitor feeling of swelling in affected limb
		Educate on the use of patient-reported outcome measures
Reports feeling of discomfort in affected limb	Decreased feeling of discomfort in affected limb	Educate on self-monitoring of discomfort in affected limb
		Monitor feeling of discomfort in affected limb
		Educate on the use of patient-reported outcome measures

Reports feeling of heaviness in affected limb	Decreased feeling of heaviness in affected limb	Educate on self-monitoring for feeling of heaviness in affected limb Monitor feeling of heaviness in affected limb
Inappropriate use of compression garments	Appropriate use of compression garments	Educate on proper use of compression garments Educate on importance of proper use of compression garments
Inattentive to carrying heavy objects	Attentive to carrying heavy objects	Educate on the consequences of carrying heavy objects
Reduced range of motion of affected limb	Improved range of motion of affected limb	Educate on self-monitoring of range of motion Monitor range of motion Educate on maintenance of motor activity when using compressive sleeves for breast cancer-related lymphedema

4. Activity/rest

Domain 4 • Class 4 • Diagnosis Code 00281

Risk for ineffective lymphedema self-management

Edvane Birelo Lopes De Domenico, Camila Takáo Lopes

NANDA International, Inc. Nursing Diagnoses: Definitions and Classification 2021–2023, 12th Edition, p. 303

Definition
Susceptible to unsatisfactory management of symptoms, treatment regimen, physical, psychosocial and spiritual consequences and lifestyle changes inherent in living with edema related to obstruction or disorders of lymph vessels or nodes, which may compromise health.

Model case
Mrs. L.S., a 45-year-old woman, was diagnosed with advanced breast cancer and underwent a 9-month neoadjuvant antineoplastic chemotherapy. During this period, despite being warned about the risks inherent to surgery with lymph node dissection, she did not attend the pre-surgery educational support program for breast cancer, in which nurses and physical therapists educate clients on the procedure, postural corrections, and provide specific stretching and exercises aiming for better surgical recovery.

After completing the antineoplastic chemotherapy protocol, she had a total mastectomy of her right breast and axillary dissection of 25 lymph nodes. Following clinical treatment, she underwent 38 radiotherapy sessions. She was again included in the education and care program to reduce the risk of lymphedema. However, the client reported that she could not make time for multidisciplinary appointments due to having resumed her work activities. Printed educational materials were provided to the client with information about the lymphatic system, concepts of normal load versus overload, instructions on how to avoid trauma or injury, infection prevention, regular physical activity, body weight management, etc. She was offered the possibility of scheduling appointments with nurses and/or physical therapists in case of concerns, but she did not schedule any appointments.

Twelve months after the surgical procedure, she returns to an oncology medical appointment with a complaint of pain in her scapular region, swelling and hardening of the skin in her upper limb, decreased arm movement, and severe pain requiring frequent use of analgesic medication. She reports being on a leave of absence from work and not being able to perform instrumental activities of daily living, such as buying food and preparing it, and having to turn to friends to help her.

An intensive plan of care is proposed to Mrs. L.S., including health education, stretching, exercises, and a compression mechanism to prevent the progression of complications caused by lymphedema. However, Mrs. L.S. states that she feels she might not be capable of keeping up with all these measures, as her strength has been drained. She states, "lymphedema cannot be worse than the cancer itself, can it?" and reports feeling extremely angry and sad about the whole cancer treatment and states, "now this new situation won't leave me alone".

Assessment

During the assessment, the nurse collected the following data, which could be interpreted to be risk (causative/predisposing) factors for this diagnosis:
- Low self-efficacy
- Negative feelings toward treatment regimen
- Unrealistic perception of seriousness of condition

Although nurses cannot intervene upon populations who are at risk for a condition, or associated conditions, it is important to be aware of individuals for whom a nursing diagnosis might be more likely to occur. Thus, the nurse should have identified the following at risk population and associated conditions that would potentially alert the nurse to concerns for this diagnosis:
- Individuals with history of ineffective health self-management
- Chemotherapy
- Major surgery
- Neoplasms
- Removal of lymph nodes

Listed below are some examples of nursing goals, outcomes and actions, linked to etiological factors. This is not presented as a comprehensive plan of care, but rather provides examples to demonstrate the proper method for linking diagnosis to outcomes and interventions, in an evidence-based manner.

L.S.'s nursing diagnosis, ultimate goal, outcomes and nursing actions

Nursing diagnosis	Risk for ineffective lymphedema self-management (00281)	
Ultimate goal(s)	Effective lymphedema self-management	
Risk factors	**Outcomes**	**Nursing actions**
Low self-efficacy	High self-efficacy	Assist with self-regulation techniques Use verbal persuasion through motivational interviewing Assist with goal setting Promote role-modeling educational strategies Provide positive feedback on accomplishments Determine rewards for accomplishments Educate on the use of client-reported outcome measures

4. Activity/rest

4. Activity/rest

Negative feelings toward treatment regimen	Positive feelings toward treatment regime	Educate on self-evaluation and self-reinforcement Educate on the use of client-reported outcome measures Identify and include sources of social support Facilitate opportunities for vicarious experience in group discussions with other clients and family members Offer complementary/integrative health care options for mood regulation, according to belief/preference Encourage maintenance of an exercise program that includes aerobic and resistance exercise, initially supervised to ensure proper technique and progression, and reinforce that practice will not cause or worsen lymphedema.
Unrealistic perception of seriousness of condition	Realistic perception of seriousness of condition	Educate on the potential consequences of lymphedema Explain the importance of complete decongestive therapy for breast cancer related lymphedema from a certified lymphedema therapist Educate on use of case-reported outcome measures Reinforce the importance of diagnosing lymphedema at an early stage for an immediate intervention capable of reversing the process Facilitate opportunities for vicarious experience in group discussions with other clients and family members

Domain 4 • Class 4 • Diagnosis Code 00291

Risk for thrombosis

Camila Takáo Lopes, Vitor Latorre Souza

NANDA International, Inc. Nursing Diagnoses: Definitions and Classification 2021–2023, 12th Edition, p. 307

Definition
Susceptible to obstruction of a blood vessel by a thrombus that can break off and lodge in another vessel, which may compromise health.

4. Activity/rest

Model case
Mr. S.W. is 45 years old, with a history of deep vein thrombosis (DVT) seven years ago. He had a partial prostatectomy four days ago due to benign prostatic hyperplasia, and was discharged home on the first postoperative day. Because he has a history of DVT and varicose veins, he was prescribed subcutaneous Enoxaparin 40 mg/day for 14 days, and 20 mmHg compression stockings. His daughter calls the ambulatory nurse and tells her that she is worried because Mr. S.W. smokes one pack of cigarettes every two days and he is still struggling with quitting. He has always been sedentary, and although she reminds him that the healthcare providers at the hospital told them that he could walk since day two, he says that it is too soon. He is letting her apply the Enoxaparin, but has been complaining a lot about his compression stockings.

Assessment
During the assessment, the nurse collected the following data, which could be interpreted to be risk (causative/predisposing) factors for this diagnosis:
- Inadequate knowledge of modifiable factors
- Sedentary lifestyle
- Smoking

Although nurses cannot independently intervene upon at risk populations or associated conditions, it is important to be aware of individuals for whom a nursing diagnosis might be more likely to occur. Thus, the nurse should have identified the following at risk population and associated condition that would potentially alert the nurse to concerns for this diagnosis:
- Individuals with history of thrombotic disease
- Surgical procedures

Listed below are some examples of nursing goals, outcomes and actions, linked to etiological factors. This is not presented as a comprehensive plan of care, but rather provides examples to demonstrate the proper method for linking diagnosis to outcomes and interventions, in an evidence-based manner.

S.W.'s nursing diagnosis, ultimate goal, outcomes and nursing actions

Nursing diagnosis	Risk for thrombosis (00291)	
Ultimate goal(s)	Absence of thrombosis	
Risk factors	**Outcomes**	**Nursing actions**
Ineffective management of preventive measures	Adequate management of modifiable factors	Educate on modifiable risk factors for deep vein thrombosis Educate on client's high risk for postoperative thrombosis Review methods used to put compression stockings on, and correct as needed
Sedentary lifestyle	Active lifestyle	Educate on misconceptions about the recovery and rehabilitation periods Educate on walking at a brisk pace for 30 minutes for at least 5 days per week, as a short-term goal for physical activity Determine medium- and long-term goals for physical activity
Smoking	Smoking cessation	Determine state of readiness for smoking reduction (pre-contemplation, contemplation, preparation) Refer for motivational interviewing or cognitive behavior therapy focused on smoking cessation Refer to pharmacotherapy program for smoking cessation if needed Offer smoking cessation counseling Identify and provide information on support groups for individuals wanting to undertake lifestyle changes Consider use of social media and online applications to support lifestyle changes

Domain 4 • Class 4 • Diagnosis Code 00318

Dysfunctional adult ventilatory weaning response

Vinicius Batista Santos, Camila Takáo Lopes

NANDA International, Inc. Nursing Diagnoses: Definitions and Classification 2021–2023, 12th Edition, p. 314

Definition
Inability to adjust to lowered levels of mechanical ventilator support that interrupts and prolongs the weaning process.

Model case
Mr V.S., 70 years old, has GOLD II chronic obstructive pulmonary disease, and is currently hospitalized with right lower lobe pneumonia. He was admitted with significant clinical signs of respiratory failure (respiratory rate of 40 bpm, use of accessory muscles, and significant hypoxemia). Non-invasive mechanical ventilatory support was initiated, however, due to the refractoriness of the condition and a reduction in his level of consciousness, orotracheal intubation was performed. During the ICU stay, Mr. V.S. has been receiving broad-spectrum antibiotic therapy. He has been in light sedation, with irregular periods of sleep and wakefulness, about 6 hours of sleep during daytime hours and only 3 hours during the night, with frequent awakenings.

On the 7th day of hospitalization, although rhonchi remain throughout the right lung base on auscultation, a reduction in intravenous sedation and ventilatory parameters was initiated due to improvements in his radiological image, pulmonary ultrasound parameters, white blood cell count, inflammatory markers, and arterial blood gasses. However, 25 minutes after his ventilation mode was shifted to pressure support, he had a significant increase of both his heart rate and respiratory rate, with a significant reduction in his inspiratory tidal volume. His breath sounds became reduced and he presented with worsening of expiratory wheezes, scattered throughout lung fields on auscultation. He had a significant increase in the use of his intercostal muscles, and a drop in his oxygen saturation (85%), accompanied by psychomotor agitation. Light sedation was resumed, his ventilation mode was shifted back to assisted-controlled and his FiO_2 was optimized.

Assessment
During the assessment, the nurse collected the following data, which could be interpreted to be related (causative) factors for this diagnosis:
– Excessive airway secretions
– Altered sleep-wake cycle

The nurse also collected the following data, which would be interpreted as defining characteristics for this diagnosis:
- Psychomotor agitation
- Increased heart rate (> 140 bpm or > 20% from baseline)
- Increased respiratory rate (> 35 rpm or > 50% over baseline)
- Decreased oxygen saturation (< 90% when fraction of inspired oxygen ratio > 40%)
- Uses significant respiratory accessory muscles
- Adventitious breath sounds

Although nurses cannot independently intervene upon at risk populations or associated conditions, it is important to be aware of individuals for whom a nursing diagnosis might be more likely to occur. Thus, the nurse should have identified the following associated condition that would potentially alert the nurse to concerns for this diagnosis:
- High acuity illness

Listed below are some examples of nursing goals, outcomes and actions, primarily linked to etiological factors. This is not presented as a comprehensive plan of care, but rather provides examples to demonstrate the proper method for linking diagnosis to outcomes and interventions, in an evidence-based manner.

V.S.'s nursing diagnosis, ultimate goal, outcomes and nursing actions

Nursing diagnosis	Dysfunctional adult ventilatory weaning response (00318)	
Ultimate goal(s)	Functional adult ventilatory weaning response	
Related factors	**Outcomes**	**Nursing actions**
Excessive airway secretions	Reduction of airway secretions	Aspirate airway as needed
Altered sleep-wake cycle	Improved sleep-wake cycle	Implement noise reduction measures Promote systematic quiet periods and dim room lights Implement measures to promote a natural circadian rhythm Ensure adequate pain management Cluster nursing care activities at night
Defining characteristics	**Outcomes**	**Nursing actions**
Psychomotor agitation	Psychomotor comfort	Monitor for psychomotor agitation
Uses significant respiratory accessory muscles	Unlabored breathing	Monitor for the use of respiratory accessory muscles Maintain head of bed elevated
Adventitious breath sounds	Decrease in adventitious breath sounds Absence of adventitious breath sounds	Monitor for adventitious breath sounds

Domain 5.
Perception/cognition

Class 4.	Cognition	
Code	Diagnosis	Page
00279	Disturbed thought process	102

Domain 5 • Class 4 • Diagnosis Code 00279

Disturbed thought process

Thiago da Silva Domingos, Camila Takáo Lopes

NANDA International, Inc. Nursing Diagnoses: Definitions and Classification 2021–2023, 12th Edition, p. 334

Definition
Disruption in cognitive functioning that affects the mental processes involved in developing concepts and categories, reasoning, and problem solving.

Model case*
Mrs. T.F. is a 45-year-old woman who lives with her 32-year-old daughter, with whom she has a strong and harmonious relationship. Mrs. T.F. is being evaluated by the nurse at her home, because she has been hearing voices telling her that she must kill herself with a knife, and that her neighbors want to hurt her.

Mrs. T.F. informs the nurse that she believes that the voices are real, so she tries to tell them to go away, closes her eyes, says a prayer, and covers her face with a pillow. She has been diagnosed with borderline personality disorder, but she says she does not trust healthcare professionals because, "all they want is to give you lots and lots of these mean pills, and I keep hearing the voices".

During the day, she tries to take care of her household chores, which makes the voices move away from her. Mrs. T.F. is a religious person and says that "only God can take someone's life". When the voices talk to her, she thinks about her daughter. She claims to be afraid though, because she doesn't know how long she will have control to ignore the voices.

Mrs. T.F. has also been having visual hallucinations, which she describes as "an older woman, who comes to my bedroom at night and gives me a knife". She shows up at night because "she is busy visiting other people" and she enters their house "because she found our key under the doormat".

T.F. reports having left the biological father of her child to live with another partner nine years ago. She mentions that her new partner was a store burglar, and that she also robbed stores for a period. She was in prison for one year for burglary and then three years for drug dealing. She says she feels guilty about her past: "I got involved with the wrong person, I ended my life there".

* Adapted from: Domingos TS, Sousa GS, Honorato TG, Oliveira JC. Distúrbio no processo de pensamento: importante diagnóstico para o cuidado de enfermagem em saúde mental. In: NANDA International, Inc.; Herdman TH, Napoleão AA, Lopes CT, Silva VM, organizadoras. PRONANDA Programa de Atualização em Diagnósticos de Enfermagem: Ciclo 10. Porto Alegre: Artmed Panamericana; 2022. p. 113–53. (Sistema de Educação Continuada a Distância, v. 2). https://doi.org/10.5935/978–65–5848–619–0.C0003 with permission from Grupo A, Artmed.

After leaving prison, she feels anguish, hatred, a very strong chest tightness and a lump in her throat. She expresses a "willingness to break everything", as she believes she can no longer bear the anguish, sadness, or auditory and visual hallucinations.

T.F. craves affection. She says, "no one in my family talks to me because I was in prison". She feels abandoned, with the exception of her daughter. As she says this, she begins to cry, saying she is a "burden to her daughter" because she is not able to help her financially. She mentions a desire to get better, and her main motivation is to be able to help her daughter financially.

She refers to feeling "done". She agrees to do the activities proposed by her daughter, such as having her nails painted and hair done, but these activities do not give her pleasure. Her self-esteem appears to be weakened.

She wears clothes that are suitable for the temperature and environment, her appearance and hygiene are good. The woman has a childish, cooperative, and receptive attitude towards the nurse. She is alert, autopsychically oriented, but allopsychically disoriented. In addition, she has a hypothymic mood; a congruent, resonant, hypomodulated affect, with apparent anhedonia and periods of anxiety and distress. The form and content of her thinking are appropriate, and no thought disturbances are noted.

Assessment

During the assessment, the nurse collected the following data, which could be interpreted to be related (causative) factors for this diagnosis:
- Anxiety
- Fear
- Non-psychotic depressive symptoms
- Stressors
- Unaddressed trauma

The nurse also collected the following data, which would be interpreted as defining characteristics for this diagnosis:
- Disorganized thought sequence
- Expresses unreal thoughts
- Impaired interpretation of events
- Impaired judgment
- Inadequate emotional response to situations
- Limited ability to perform expected social roles
- Limited ability to plan activities
- Limited impulse control ability
- Phobic disorders
- Suspicions
- Hallucinations

Listed below are some examples of nursing goals, outcomes and actions, primarily linked to etiological factors. This is not presented as a comprehensive plan of care, but rather provides examples to demonstrate the proper method for linking diagnosis to outcomes and interventions, in an evidence-based manner.

T.F.'s nursing diagnosis, ultimate goal, outcomes and nursing actions

Nursing diagnosis	Disturbed thought process (00279)	
Ultimate goal(s)	Self-management of disturbed thoughts	
Related factors	Outcomes	Nursing actions
Anxiety	Decreased anxiety level Increased tranquility level	Support in identifying anxiety-triggering situations. Implement anxiety-reducing strategies Approach in a slow, calm, matter-of-fact manner Listen attentively to feelings, perceptions, and experiences
Fear	Identification of feelings, perceptions, and emotions related to situations of fear Decreased level of fear	Establish rapport Support in identifying fear-triggering situations Assure the client of her safety and security by not leaving her alone while experiencing symptoms
Non-psychotic depressive symptoms	Decreased level of depressive symptoms	Demonstrate acceptance and understanding of the depressive symptoms Provide a nonjudgmental approach while preserving confidentiality Use silence and active listening during interactions Monitor severity of depressive symptoms using a standardized tool Let client know that you are concerned and that her feelings matter Refer to specialized psychological care, as needed
Stressors	Stressor self-management	Support the use of appropriate defense mechanisms Decrease environmental stimuli as much as possible Assess for successful coping strategies used in the past
Unaddressed trauma	Trauma elaboration	Assist with coping strategies Listen attentively to feelings, perceptions, and experiences Show empathy regarding feelings

Defining characteristics	Outcomes	Nursing actions
Disorganized thought sequence	Organized thought process	Monitor organization of thought sequence Use simple, concrete, or direct messages, and avoid use of abstractions Assist continuously with ability to think logically and in an organized way
Expresses unreal thoughts	Interacts on reality-based topics	Refrain from pursuing the details of hallucinations, or challenging the hallucination system Do not validate delusional ideas Acknowledge feelings are real, but delusional ideas are not real
Limited impulse control ability	Improved impulse control ability	Monitor intention to obey auditory hallucinations Make a list of challenging situations with client Establish a set of assertive approaches to the situations Encourage to select an approach and make specific plans for implementation Teach about assertive skills and how to differentiate passive, aggressive, and assertive responses
Suspicions	Trust in established relationships	Introduce client to each healthcare provider Refrain from making promises that cannot be kept Ensure procedures are understood before performing them

5. Perception/cognition

Domain 7.
Role relationship

Class 2.	Family relationships	
Code	**Diagnosis**	**Page**
00283	Disturbed family identity syndrome	108
00284	Risk for disturbed family identity syndrome	111

Domain 7 • Class 2 • Diagnosis Code 00283

Disturbed family identity syndrome

Anneliese Domingues Wysocki, Andreia Cascaez Cruz, Camila Takáo Lopes

NANDA International, Inc. Nursing Diagnoses: Definitions and Classification 2021–2023, 12th Edition, p. 370

Definition
Inability to maintain an ongoing interactive, communicative process of creating and maintaining a shared collective sense of the meaning of the family.

Model case*
Mrs. H.R., a 40-year-old supermarket manager, was divorced after 16 years and has two children: A.R. is 12, and F.R. is 14 years of age. Four years after her divorce Mrs. H.R. married Mr. E.P., six months ago, and she and her children moved into his house. E.P. is a 42-year-old mechanic who had never been married and has no children. Before moving in together, the family members were very supportive of each other. The four of them had dinner together at the table every weekend and discussed about their weekly routines.

After moving in, Mrs. H.R. has been arguing with Mr. E.P. daily about their different responses to behavioral issues of the children, and it gets worse every day. He disagrees with the children eating while watching TV, staying up late, and their screen time on their phones or video gaming. The children used to like Mr. E.P. before moving in, but now they refuse to talk to him, except to offend him. They don't spend time together anymore and stopped talking about their everyday routine. A.R. has been exhibiting poor school performance and F.R. has been isolating himself. Mrs. H.R. feels tense and guilty all the time, cannot concentrate at work, and has been having several arguments with colleagues, which rarely ever happened previously.. She is unsure how to handle the family disagreements, and whenever her children try to talk to her about the situation at home, she avoids them. She says she strange and says she doesn't recognize herself anymore.

Assessment
During the assessment, the nurse collected the following data, which could be interpreted to be related (causative) factors for this diagnosis:
- Different coping styles among family members
- Disrupted family rituals

* Adapted from: Herdman, T.H., Jones, D.A., Lopes, C.T. Clinical Application: Data Analysis to Determine Appropriate Nursing Diagnosis. In: Herdman, T.H., Kamitsuru, S., Lopes, C.T. (2021). NANDA International nursing diagnoses: definitions and classification, 2021–2023. Thieme Publishers. New York. pp. 126–137.

- Ineffective family communication
- Excessive stress

The nurse also collected the following data, which would be interpreted as defining characteristics for this diagnosis:

Disturbed personal identity (00121)
- Expresses feeling of strangeness
- Inadequate interpersonal relations
- Inadequate role performance
- Ineffective coping strategies

Dysfunctional family processes (00063)
- Difficulty adapting to change
- Escalating conflict

Ineffective relationship (00223)
- Delayed attainment of developmental goals appropriate for family life-cycle stage
- Partner not identified as support person
- Reports unsatisfactory communication with partner

Interrupted family processes (00060)
- Decreased mutual support
- Altered family conflict resolution
- Altered communication pattern

Although nurses cannot independently intervene upon at risk populations or associated conditions, it is important to be aware of individuals for whom a nursing diagnosis might be more likely to occur. Thus, the nurse should have identified the following at risk populations that would potentially alert the nurse to concerns for this diagnosis:

- Blended families
- Different coping styles among family members
- Disrupted family rituals
- Ineffective family communication

Listed below are some examples of nursing goals, outcomes and actions, primarily linked to etiological factors. This is not presented as a comprehensive plan of care, but rather provides examples to demonstrate the proper method for linking diagnosis to outcomes and interventions, in an evidence-based manner.

7. Role relationship

H.R.'s family nursing diagnosis, ultimate goal, outcomes and nursing actions

Nursing diagnosis	Disturbed family identity syndrome (00283)	
Ultimate goal(s)	Preserved family identity	

Related factors	Outcomes	Nursing actions
Different coping styles among family members	Improved family coping	Recognize family's expectations of functioning
Disrupted family rituals	Organized family rituals	Promote dialogue about the new family configuration
Ineffective family communication	Effective family communication	Discuss developmental goals for current family life-cycle stage
Excessive stress	Decreased stress	Promote dialogue about couple's expectation of family life
		Promote dialogue about children's expectations of the new family life
		Promote dialogue about stepfather's expectations of the relationship with the children
		Clarify the roles of family members
		Assist family in developing family rituals
		Assist children and parents in dealing with fears and conflicts related to the family
		Assist family in negotiating rules and household chores
		Outline coping strategies with the family
		Educate on strategies for stress relief

Defining characteristics	Outcomes	Nursing actions
Disturbed personal identity (00121)	Organized personal identity	Monitor interpersonal relations
Dysfunctional family processes (00063)	Functional family processes	Monitor role performance
Interrupted family processes (00060)	Uninterrupted family processes	Monitor coping strategies
Ineffective relationship (00223)	Effective relationship	Monitor adaptation to change
		Educate on positive ways to resolve conflict,
		Educate on self-monitoring of attainment of developmental goals for family life-cycle stage
		Monitor for sense of mutual partner support
		Monitor satisfaction with communication with partner
		Monitor for communication pattern

Domain 7 • Class 2 • Diagnosis Code 00284

Risk for disturbed family identity syndrome

Andreia Cascaez Cruz, Anneliese Domingues Wysocki, Camila Takáo Lopes

NANDA International, Inc. Nursing Diagnoses: Definitions and Classification 2021–2023, 12th Edition, p. 372

> **Definition**
> Susceptible to an inability to maintain an ongoing interactive, communicative process of creating and maintaining a shared collective sense of the meaning of the family, which may compromise family members' health.

Model case

Mrs. F.J., a 32-year-old saleswoman, and Mr. I.J., a 36-year-old engineer, have been married for four years. They had been trying to get pregnant for 18 months when she was diagnosed with tubal infertility, and he was diagnosed with oligozoospermia. An in vitro fertilization (IVF) with intracytoplasmic sperm injection was indicated as a treatment. Both were anxious about the treatment and had expectations of family support.

One week ago, at a family gathering, they told their parents that they intended to follow through with the treatment in another city, where there was a specialized clinic and a strong record of positive results. Mr. I.J.'s mother told them that they should not have this type of treatment, because it was unnatural. She believed that there was a problem with Mrs. F.J. because women are not supposed to have jobs other than in the home, and she was sure that they would soon get pregnant if she stopped working. Mrs. F.J.'s parents then got into an argument with her, and left the house.

Since then, the couple have not talked to their parents or even talked with one another about the issue. Mrs. F.J. has been upset the whole week, barely speaking to her husband because he did not disagree with what his mother said.

Assessment

During the assessment, the nurse collected the following data, which could be interpreted to be risk (causative/predisposing) factors for this diagnosis:
- Inadequate social support
- Ineffective family communication
- Values incongruent with cultural norms

Although nurses cannot independently intervene upon at risk populations or associated conditions, it is important to be aware of individuals for whom a nursing diagnosis might be more likely to occur. Thus, the nurse should have

7. Role relationship

identified the following at risk populations that would potentially alert the nurse to concerns for this diagnosis:
- Families experiencing infertility

Listed below are some examples of nursing goals, outcomes and actions, linked to etiological factors. This is not presented as a comprehensive plan of care, but rather provides examples to demonstrate the proper method for linking diagnosis to outcomes and interventions, in an evidence-based manner.

F.J.'s and I.J.'s family nursing diagnosis, ultimate goal, outcomes and nursing actions

Nursing diagnosis	Risk for disturbed family identity syndrome (00284)	
Ultimate goal(s)	Preserved family identity	
Risk factors	**Outcomes**	**Nursing actions**
Inadequate social support	Adequate social support	Identify and include sources of social support
Ineffective family communication	Effective family communication	Identify and provide information on support groups providing local or online support to individuals with infertility
Values incongruent with cultural norms	Respect for each other's values	Outline communication strategies with the family
		Promote dialogue among family members about infertility and in vitro fertilization
		Assess and discuss the couple's expectation about their family role regarding their decision about in vitro fertilization
		Assist the couple to understand their role regarding their nuclear family and their parents
		Assist the couple to negotiate boundaries regarding their parents

Domain 9.
Coping/stress tolerance

Class 2. Coping responses

Code	Diagnosis	Page
00301	Maladaptive grieving	114
00302	Risk for maladaptive grieving	116
00285	Readiness for enhanced grieving	119

Domain 9 • Class 2 • Diagnosis Code 00301

Maladaptive grieving

T. Heather Herdman

NANDA International, Inc. Nursing Diagnoses: Definitions and Classification 2021–2023, 12th Edition, p. 421

Definition
A disorder that occurs after the death of a significant other, in which the experience of distress accompanying bereavement fails to follow sociocultural expectations.

Model case
W.P. is a 23-year-old woman who lost her father 13 months ago in a traumatic car accident, when he apparently fell asleep while driving and his car ran off the road, flipped down a hill, and crashed into some trees. Their relationship had been incredibly close, as he was her only living family, and she saw him as her primary source of support. W.P. is unmarried and states she has few close friends. Her mother died from cancer when she was three years old.

W.P. was fired from her job six months ago due to lack of attendance and not providing notice of absences, which has left her in an economically unstable condition. She seems very nervous about this situation but says she cannot do anything about it right now, her grief is her priority, so she just can't cope with this issue right now.

She began attending a support group for bereaved relatives three months ago, and she was referred for follow up because of concerns regarding her health. When she came to see the nurse, her appearance was unkempt and she did not appear to be maintaining her bodily hygiene. While talking with the community health nurse, W.P. notes that she has consistent nightmares about the accident that killed her father. She finds herself thinking about how her father must have felt as he was in the middle of the accident, which triggers an overwhelming feeling of fear and panic.

W.P. tells the nurse that her few friends and even people in the support group seem to value her loss less than that of a spouse or child, because those are considered worse than the death of a parent. When she tried to talk with them about her father, she felt they always wanted to change the subject, so she lost trust in people. This has led her to withdraw from social interactions which she finds unsupportive, leaving her with more time to obsess about and long for time with her father. Today she tells the nurses that she feels numb, empty, and disconnected from her life before the accident.

Assessment

During the assessment, the nurse would have collected the following data, which could be interpreted to be related factors for this diagnosis:
- Difficulty dealing with concurrent crises
- Inadequate social support

The nurse also collected the following data, which would be interpreted as defining characteristics for this diagnosis:
- Decreased life role performance
- Depressive symptoms
- Expresses distress about the deceased person
- Expresses feeling detached from others
- Expresses feeling of emptiness
- Mistrust of others
- Preoccupation with thoughts about the deceased person
- Rumination about the deceased person

Although nurses cannot independently intervene upon at risk populations or associated conditions, it is important to be aware of individuals for whom a nursing diagnosis might be more likely to occur. Thus, the nurse should have identified the following at risk populations that would potentially alert the nurse to concerns for this diagnosis:
- Individuals experiencing unexpected sudden loss of significant other
- Individuals experiencing violent death of significant other
- Individuals with strong emotional proximity to the deceased
- Women

Listed below are some examples of nursing goals, outcomes and actions, primarily linked to etiological factors. This is not presented as a comprehensive plan of care, but rather provides examples to demonstrate the proper method for linking diagnosis to outcomes and interventions, in an evidence-based manner.

W.P.'s nursing diagnosis, ultimate goal, outcomes and nursing actions

Nursing diagnosis	Maladaptive grieving (00301)	
Ultimate goal(s)	Healthy grieving	
Related factors	Outcomes	Nursing actions
Inadequate social support	Adequate social support	Identify and include sources of social support Encourage continuation with support group for individuals who are grieving Counsel on methods to decrease interpersonal stress
Difficulty dealing with concurrent crises	Ability to cope with concurrent crises	Target avoidance behavior using Complicated Grief Therapy Encourage repeated telling of the story of learning of the death Focus on understanding the loss in the context of the client's biography Introduce daily grief monitoring Begin aspirational goal setting

9. Coping/stress tolerance

Domain 9 • Class 2 • Diagnosis Code 00302

Risk for maladaptive grieving

T. Heather Herdman

NANDA International, Inc. Nursing Diagnoses: Definitions and Classification 2021–2023, 12th Edition, p. 423

Definition
Susceptible to a disorder that occurs after the death of a significant other, in which the experience of distress accompanying bereavement fails to follow sociocultural expectations, which may compromise health.

Model case
T.M. is a 60-year-old woman who recently lost her mother, who was 91 years of age and had been living with her for approximately two years prior to her death. Their relationship was very difficult throughout most of T.M.'s life, with significant conflict whenever T.M. made decisions that weren't approved of by her mother. However, in the past two years the two became much closer, spending time talking, enjoying cultural events, eating out when possible, and sharing time watching TV or talking about books they had read.

In a regular check-up visit for an autoimmune condition she has been managing for several years, T.M. began crying when the nurse asked how she was doing after her mother's death, which was 4 months ago. She indicated she had been having a lot of difficulty sleeping and finally asked her doctor for sleeping pills, which she has been taking regularly but without much success. She finds herself unable to control her emotions, and flips from happiness to anger or sadness without any warning. She finds herself crying almost every day, and this is very odd behavior for her, she says. She indicates she has been very curt with some friends and her boss even spoke with her about her "outbursts" of inappropriate anger at work the other day. She has been finding it difficult to concentrate, has little interest in food, and has stopped her normal physical exercise routine because she simply has no motivation.

T.M. notes that it was incredibly difficult to watch her mother, a very strong and determined woman, become disabled so quickly. The most difficult thing for her was to observe her episodes of extreme fear, which seemed to occur without warning and lasted for long periods of time. Her mother was experiencing visual and auditory hallucinations, and the hospice team hadn't been able to address these. T.M. was blaming herself for not dealing better with these symptoms and reacting by medicating her mother so she would sleep because she couldn't handle seeing her in this way.

After further discussion, T.M. acknowledges she was always a little afraid of her mother, because her moods had been quick to change when she was a child, and she often felt she bore the brunt of her mother's anger. Even as an adult, she found it hard to disagree openly with her mother for fear of her response. Now she says she wishes she had been strong enough to talk about the way she felt and resolve this conflict while her mother was still alive. She also wishes she had taken more time to talk with her in depth about how her mother wanted to handle end of life care, although they had some general discussion.

T.M. notes that it is strange to her to realize how much she misses her mother now that she is gone, and how she longs to tell her things she has seen or done during her day, and to ask her more questions about her life that she can now never ask her. She also indicates that her closest friends have also lost a parent recently and they do not want to talk about how she feels, and they both seem much more at peace than she feels herself.

Assessment

During the assessment, the nurse collected the following data, which could be interpreted to be risk (causative/predisposing) factors for this diagnosis:
- Excessive emotional disturbance
- Inadequate social support

Although nurses cannot independently intervene upon at risk populations or associated conditions, it is important to be aware of individuals for whom a nursing diagnosis might be more likely to occur. Thus, the nurse should have identified the following at risk populations that would potentially alert the nurse to concerns for this diagnosis:
- Individuals with strong emotional proximity to the deceased
- Individuals who witnessed uncontrolled symptoms of the deceased
- Individuals with unresolved conflict with the deceased

Listed below are some examples of nursing goals, outcomes and actions, linked to etiological factors. This is not presented as a comprehensive plan of care, but rather provides examples to demonstrate the proper method for linking diagnosis to outcomes and interventions, in an evidence-based manner.

9. Coping/stress tolerance

W.P.'s nursing diagnosis, ultimate goal, outcomes and nursing actions

Nursing diagnosis	Risk for maladaptive grieving (00302)	
Ultimate goal(s)	Healthy grieving	
Risk factors	**Outcomes**	**Nursing actions**
Excessive emotional disturbance	Emotional stability	Consider cognitive behavioral therapy Provide education regarding cognitive restructuring and stimulus control Train to use relaxation techniques Identify and provide information on support groups providing local or online support to individuals dealing with loss of a significant other Refer for psychological evaluation and follow-up, as needed Encourage engagement in mindfulness practices to develop self-awareness
Inadequate social support	Adequate social support	Identify and include current sources of social support Counsel on methods to decrease interpersonal stress Encourage client to reach out to other sources of support within her network Refer for spiritual guidance, if desired

Domain 9 • Class 2 • Diagnosis Code 00285

Readiness for enhanced grieving

T. Heather Herdman

NANDA International, Inc. Nursing Diagnoses: Definitions and Classification 2021–2023, 12th Edition, p. 424

Definition
A pattern of integration of a new functional reality that arises after an actual, anticipated or perceived significant loss, which can be strengthened.

Model case
H.M. is a 34-year-old man who has recently lost his mother after a long course of treatment for melanoma. He indicates that he knows she is no longer suffering, which gives him great comfort, but he had never really allowed himself to believe she would die. He now finds himself grieving her death more acutely than he expected. His partner is very supportive, and recommended he attend a support group, but he isn't a very gregarious individual and wanted to meet with an individual grief counselor first. As his hospice support nurse, Nurse Celia meets with him to discuss how he is doing.

H.M. says he wants his mother's life to be more important than her death, and he wants to incorporate the positive memories with his mother into his life as he moves forward, because he feels this would be a good tribute to her influence on him. He says he wants to be able to acknowledge his loss and integrate it into his life, not ignoring it, but also not letting it take control of his life. Ultimately he wants to use her death to remind him what is important to him, and to put more energy into his remaining significant relationships, and "find his joy".

Assessment
During the assessment, the nurse collected the following data, which would be interpreted as defining characteristics of motivation and desire to increase well-being and to actualize health potential:
- Expresses desire to integrate positive memories of the deceased
- Expresses desire to integrate possibilities for a joyful life
- Expresses desire to integrate the loss

Listed below are some examples of nursing goals, outcomes and actions, primarily linked to etiological factors. This is not presented as a comprehensive plan of care, but rather provides examples to demonstrate the proper method for linking diagnosis to outcomes and interventions, in an evidence-based manner.

H.M.'s nursing diagnosis, ultimate goal, outcomes and nursing actions

Nursing diagnosis	Readiness for enhanced grieving (00285)	
Ultimate goal(s)	Enhanced grieving	
Defining characteristics	**Outcomes**	**Nursing actions**
Expresses desire to integrate positive memories of the deceased	Integration of positive memories of the deceased	Encourage journaling positive memories of deceased Encourage sharing positive stories about deceased Facilitate client's practice of self-compassion
Expresses desire to integrate the loss	Integration of the loss	Support client in making meaning of the death Support client in regaining a positive, hopeful outlook that supports active agency Support client's resilience Encourage engagement in mindfulness practices to develop self-awareness
Expresses desire to integrate possibilities for a joyful life	Integration of possibilities for a joyful life	Support in mastering the possible and holding hope in future possibilities with sustained effort Support spiritual dimension of loss experience Find creative ways to celebrate important events, incorporating loss into new positive experiences

Domain 11.
Safety/protection

Class 2. Physical injury

Code	Diagnosis	Page
00277	Ineffective dry eye self-management	122
00303	Risk for adult falls	125
00306	Risk for child falls	128
00320	Nipple-areolar complex injury	130
00321	Risk for nipple-areolar complex injury	132
00312	Adult pressure injury	134
00304	Risk for adult pressure injury	137
00313	Child pressure injury	140
00286	Risk for child pressure injury	143
00287	Neonatal pressure injury	146
00288	Risk for neonatal pressure injury	149

Class 3. Violence

Code	Diagnosis	Page
00289	Risk for suicidal behavior	152

Class 6. Thermoregulation

Code	Diagnosis	Page
00280	Neonatal hypothermia	154
00282	Risk for neonatal hypothermia	158

Domain 11 • Class 2 • Diagnosis Code 00277

Ineffective dry eye self-management

Alexia Louisie Pontes Gonçalves, Camila Takáo Lopes

NANDA International, Inc. Nursing Diagnoses: Definitions and Classification 2021–2023, 12th Edition, p. 473

> **Definition**
> Unsatisfactory management of symptoms, treatment regimen, physical, psychosocial, and spiritual consequences and lifestyle changes inherent in living with inadequate tear film.

Model case

T.J. is a 16-year-old high school student who has been online gaming for the previous five years. He also spent the last two years in online classes due to the COVID-19 pandemic. To participate in competitions, he has been staying awake at night with a fan blowing on his face constantly for the previous three months. He drinks a lot of espresso coffee to stay awake, but he forgets to drink water, and rarely takes out his contact lenses when he finally goes to sleep. During this period, he frequently noted that his eyes were red and fatigued, and his vision was blurred. After a lot of insistence, he had an appointment with a primary healthcare nurse who explained to him that his tear film was being negatively impacted by his routine. The nurse also explained that to avoid impairing his eye, he would have to make many changes: limit his screen time, take eye breaks, perform blinking exercises when using screens, adjust the screen angle so it would be below his vision line, decrease his caffeine consumption, sleep more, remove his contact lenses for sleep, and place the fan away from his face.

T.J. has never had to make decisions about health issues before. He downplays the seriousness of his condition and thinks the nurse is overreacting because everyone has red, tired eyes from time to time. He did not tell her that, because she didn't directly ask him about his perceptions. He does not know where to start with everything that nurse Janice recommended, because she provided so much information, and he does not think he has time for all of that! He has an important online competition coming up, so he simply bought the cheapest eye drops he could find to alleviate his eye tiredness, as he was sure this would soon go away.

During the next three months, T.J. maintained all of his regular habits he had discussed with the nurse, his conjunctival hyperemia remained, but he also started feeling his eyes get more dry, they started burning and itching, and sometimes it feels as if there is sand in his eyes. He goes for help again only when he can no longer tolerate his symptoms.

Assessment

During the assessment, the nurse collected the following data, which could be interpreted to be related (causative) factors for this diagnosis:
-   Difficulty with decision-making
-   Unrealistic perception of seriousness of condition
-   Difficulty managing complex treatment regimen
-   Inadequate health literacy
-   Competing demands
-   Competing lifestyle preferences

The nurse also collected the following data, which would be interpreted as defining characteristics for this diagnosis:

Behaviors
-   Difficulty reducing caffeine consumption
-   Inappropriate use of contact lenses
-   Inappropriate use of fans
-   Inattentive to dry eye signs
-   Inattentive to dry eye symptoms
-   Insufficient fluid intake
-   Nonadherence to recommended blinking exercises
-   Nonadherence to recommended eye breaks
-   Use of products with benzalkonium chloride preservatives

Dry Eye Symptoms
-   Reports blurred vision
-   Reports eye fatigue
-   Reports feeling of burning eyes
-   Reports feeling of ocular dryness
-   Reports feeling of ocular foreign body
-   Reports feeling of ocular itching
-   Reports feeling of sand in eye

Dry Eye Signs
-   Conjunctival hyperemia

Although nurses cannot independently intervene upon at risk populations or associated conditions, it is important to be aware of individuals for whom a nursing diagnosis might be more likely to occur. Thus, the nurse should have identified the following at risk population that would potentially alert the nurse to concerns for this diagnosis:
-   Individuals with limited decision-making experience

Listed below are some examples of nursing goals, outcomes and actions, primarily linked to etiological factors. This is not presented as a comprehensive plan of care, but rather provides examples to demonstrate the proper method for linking diagnosis to outcomes and interventions, in an evidence-based manner.

T.J.'s nursing diagnosis, ultimate goal, outcomes and nursing actions

Nursing diagnosis	Ineffective dry eye self-management (00277)	
Ultimate goal(s)	Effective dry eye self-management	
Related factors	**Outcomes**	**Nursing actions**
Difficulty with decision-making	Commitment to informed decision-making	Involve client in shared decision-making
Unrealistic perception of seriousness of condition	Realistic perception of seriousness of condition	Explain and illustrate seriousness of condition
Difficulty managing complex treatment regimen	Ability to manage treatment regimen	Assist with written weekly plan strategies to manage dry eye treatment regimen
Inadequate health literacy	Adequate health literacy	Use plain language, visual aids, smartphone-based solutions, and open-ended questions, and teach-back, show-back techniques
Competing demands	Prioritizing of competing demands	Assist with prioritizing of competing demands
Competing lifestyle preferences	Prioritizing lifestyle preferences	Assist with prioritizing of lifestyle preferences
Defining characteristics	**Outcomes**	**Nursing actions**
Inattentive to dry eye signs	Attentive to dry eye signs	Educate on self-monitoring of disease signs Monitor severity of disease signs
Inattentive to dry eye symptoms	Attentive to dry eye symptoms	Educate on self-monitoring of disease symptoms Monitor severity of disease symptoms

Domain 11 • Class 2 • Diagnosis Code 00303

Risk for adult falls

T. Heather Herdman

NANDA International, Inc. Nursing Diagnoses: Definitions and Classification 2021–2023, 12th Edition, p. 476

> **Definition**
> Adult susceptible to experiencing an event resulting in coming to rest inadvertently on the ground, floor, or other lower level, which may compromise health.

Model case

N.M. is a 75-year-old widow who lives in a house with her daughter, her son-in-law,, and her granddaughters. She is completely independent for activities of daily living, but walks with a cane after having broken her hip 2 years ago. At that time she was found to have significant osteoporosis which caused her hip to shatter. She had surgical hip fracture repair with internal fixation performed after her fall, and has recovered very well. She also has mild hypertension, and a history of migraines.

At her annual exam, she was evaluated using the Falls Efficacy Scale International, and scored 76/100, indicating a fear of falling. During the discussion of the scale interpretation, N.M. tells her nurse that she had noticed in the past year that her balance is not as good as it used to be, and she finds it difficult to reach above her head without holding on to something with the other hand. She also finds going up and down stairs more difficult. She acknowledges that getting up from a chair has become harder for her. She does walk every day with her teenage granddaughters when the weather is good, which she finds helps with her stiffness. Her laboratory values indicate that she has a moderate Vitamin D deficiency, along with being deficient in Vitamin B12 and exhibiting mild anemia.

Upon further evaluation N.M. indicates that the toilet seat is quite low, and there are no safety bars to assist her in standing, nor are there safety bars in the shower, so she only takes sponge baths, because she is afraid of slipping in the shower.

Assessment

During the assessment, the nurse collected the following data, which could be interpreted to be risk (causative/predisposing) factors for this diagnosis:
- Decreased lower extremity strength
- Impaired physical mobility
- Impaired postural balance

- Vitamin D deficiency
- Fear of falling
- Inappropriate toilet seat height
- Lack of safety rails
- Factors identified by standardized, validated screening tool

Although nurses cannot independently intervene upon at risk populations or associated conditions, it is important to be aware of individuals for whom a nursing diagnosis might be more likely to occur. Thus, the nurse should have identified the following at risk populations and associated conditions that would potentially alert the nurse to concerns for this diagnosis:

- Individuals aged > 60 years
- Anemia
- Assistive devices for walking
- Musculoskeletal diseases

Listed below are some examples of nursing goals, outcomes and actions, linked to etiological factors. This is not presented as a comprehensive plan of care, but rather provides examples to demonstrate the proper method for linking diagnosis to outcomes and interventions, in an evidence-based manner.

N.M.'s nursing diagnosis, ultimate goal, outcomes and nursing actions

Nursing diagnosis	Risk for adult falls (00303)	
Ultimate goal(s)	Absence of falls	
Risk factors	**Outcomes**	**Nursing actions**
Decreased lower extremity strength	Adequate lower extremity strength	Institute program of strength training Encourage practicing moving from sitting to standing position, using safety measures, to strengthen leg muscles
Impaired physical mobility	Adequate physical mobility	Conduct environmental assessment of the home Encourage self-directed behaviors focused on physical condition Initiate progressive competency-based exercise program Perform directed-by-other mobility activities focused on physical condition Encourage increased ambulation as tolerated Teach and monitor progress with muscle strengthening exercises
Impaired postural balance	Adequate postural balance	Implement plan for balance improvement Encourage physical activity to encourage balance and avert falls at least 3x/week

Vitamin D deficiency	Normal Vitamin D levels	Educate on foods with high levels of Vitamin D Consider Vitamin D therapy 700 IU/d to 1000 IU/d for improved muscle strength and balance
Fear of falling	Decreased fear of falling	Educate client on home safety needs Teach and reinforce home safety skills
Inappropriate toilet seat height Lack of safety rails	Safety measures instituted in home	Assess living space for safety, using a standardized, validated assessment tool Identify and encourage outreach to neighborhood support organizations for improving environmental safety Identify community resources for accessing safety equipment and installation Support home modifications, including grab bars, improved lighting, and raised toilet seats, to enable ease and safety of navigating home setting

Domain 11 • Class 2 • Diagnosis Code 00306

Risk for child falls

Camila Takáo Lopes, Ana Paula Dias França Guareschi

NANDA International, Inc. Nursing Diagnoses: Definitions and Classification 2021–2023, 12th Edition, p. 478

> **Definition**
> Child susceptible to experiencing an event resulting in coming to rest inadvertently on the ground, floor, or other lower level, which may compromise health.

Model case

Ms. B.V.T. is 16 years old and has dropped out of school to take care of her child. She has a 14-month-old toddler, R.T., who has been learning how to walk. During a home visitation, the nurse observes that there are three throw rugs and lots of toys around the living room, where the toddler walks around with the aid of a walker, while wearing regular socks. Her bottle is lying on the room table out of her reach, but she repeatedly attempts to reach for it. The nurse observes Ms. B.V.T. take her daughter out of the walker and place her in a bouncer seat on the table, as she prepares to get dressed in her bedroom prior to leaving the house.

Assessment

During the assessment, the nurse collected the following data, which could be interpreted to be risk (causative/predisposing) factors for this diagnosis:

Caregiver factors
– Inadequate supervision of child
– Inattentive to environmental safety
– Places child in bouncer seat on raised surfaces
– Places child in infant walkers
– Cluttered environment
– Objects out of reach
– Use of throw rugs

Other factors
– Inappropriate footwear

Although nurses cannot independently intervene upon at risk populations or associated conditions, it is important to be aware of individuals for whom a nursing diagnosis might be more likely to occur. Thus, the nurse should have identified the following at risk populations that would potentially alert the nurse to concerns for this diagnosis:
– Children born to economically disadvantaged families

- Children whose caregivers have
- low educational level
- Children with young caregivers

Listed below are some examples of nursing goals, outcomes and actions, linked to etiological factors. This is not presented as a comprehensive plan of care, but rather provides examples to demonstrate the proper method for linking diagnosis to outcomes and interventions, in an evidence-based manner.

R.T.'s nursing diagnosis, ultimate goal, outcomes and nursing actions

Nursing diagnosis	Risk for child falls (00306)	
Ultimate goal(s)	Absence of falls	
Risk factors	**Outcomes**	**Nursing actions**
Caregiver factors		
Inadequate supervision of child	Adequate supervision of child	Educate caregiver on adequate supervision of child to prevent falls
Inattentive to environmental safety	Attentive to environmental safety	Conduct environmental assessment of the home
		Educate caregiver on aspects of environmental safety to prevent falls
		Identify and encourage outreach to neighborhood support organizations for improving environmental safety
Places child in bouncer seat on raised surfaces	Places child in bouncer seat on low surfaces	Educate caregiver on appropriate placement of child in bouncer seat on low surfaces
Places child in infant walkers	Does not use infant walkers	Educate caregiver on risk of using infant walkers to the mother
Cluttered environment	Organized environment	Educate caregiver to maintain a safe, uncluttered environment
Objects out of reach	Objects under reach	Educate caregiver to place objects within reach Educate caregiver on
Use of throw rugs	Does not use throw rugs	Educate caregiver on risk of using throw rugs to the mother
Other factors		
Inappropriate footwear	Uses appropriate footwear	Educate caregiver on the use of anti-slip socks

11. Safety/protection

Domain 11 • Class 2 • Diagnosis Code 00320

Nipple-areolar complex injury

Camila Takáo Lopes, Kelly Pereira Coca

NANDA International, Inc. Nursing Diagnoses: Definitions and Classification 2021–2023, 12th Edition, p. 482

> **Definition**
> Localized damage to the nipple-areolar complex as a result of the breastfeeding process.

Model case
Mrs. A.P.O. is a 27-year-old primiparous mother who has been breastfeeding her child for five days and requested consultation from a nurse lactation consultant. Upon physical examination, the nurse finds macerated skin and fissures with scab formation and exudate on both of her nipples and areolas. She reports nipple pain of 5 on a scale of 10. She has been applying lanolin when wearing a bra to prevent the exudate from adhering to her breast pads. She was previously taught that lanolin does not help to heal wounds, so she decided to wash the lanolin off her nipple before breastfeeding. However, sometimes when she removes her breast pads, she feels that they remove the skin. She has tried multiple times to remove the scab by rubbing her nipple and areola, but she realized she is causing more damage.

Assessment
During the assessment, the nurse collected the following data, which could be interpreted to be related (causative) factors for this diagnosis:
–   Prolonged exposure to moisture
The nurse also collected the following data, which would be interpreted as defining characteristics for this diagnosis:
–   Expresses pain
–   Macerated skin
–   Disrupted skin surface
Although nurses cannot independently intervene upon at risk populations or associated conditions, it is important to be aware of individuals for whom a nursing diagnosis might be more likely to occur. Thus, the nurse should have identified the following at risk population that would potentially alert the nurse to concerns for this diagnosis:
–   Primiparous women
Listed below are some examples of nursing goals, outcomes and actions, primarily linked to etiological factors. This is not presented as a comprehensive plan of

care, but rather provides examples to demonstrate the proper method for linking diagnosis to outcomes and interventions, in an evidence-based manner.

A.P.O.'s nursing diagnosis, ultimate goal, outcomes and nursing actions

Nursing diagnosis	Nipple-areolar complex injury (00320)	
Ultimate goal(s)	Nipple-areolar complex integrity	
Related factors	**Outcomes**	**Nursing actions**
Prolonged exposure to moisture	Shortened exposure to moisture	Educate on appropriate use of breast pads Teach to optimize time without bra, wearing soft garment Teach not to use moisturizer on areola
Defining characteristics	**Outcomes**	**Nursing actions**
Expresses pain	Expresses decreased pain level Expresses absence of pain	Assess for areolar flexibility Educate on techniques to soften the areola before breastfeeding Teach to apply expressed breast milk to wound
Macerated skin Disrupted skin surface	Skin integrity	Teach to remove breast pads carefully or to soak if adhering to skin Teach not to wash lanolin from nipple–areolar complex prior to breastfeeding Teach not to debride or rub nipple Educate on cleansing and debriding application of the infant's mouth Teach to self-monitor skin integrity Teach to self-monitor pain intensity Monitor skin maceration or fissure Monitor pain intensity using a standardized scale

Domain 11 • Class 2 • Diagnosis Code 00321

Risk for nipple-areolar complex injury

Camila Takáo Lopes, Kelly Pereira Coca

NANDA International, Inc. Nursing Diagnoses: Definitions and Classification 2021–2023, 12th Edition, p. 484

> **Definition**
> Susceptible to localized damage to nipple-areolar complex as a result of the breastfeeding process.

Model case
Ms. D.Y. is a 16-year-old, primiparous, single mother, who has been breastfeeding for two days. During assessment, the nurse finds that she has been using hand sanitizer on a cotton ball to clean her nipples between each breastfeeding because she was afraid of infections. She has been supporting her breast with a V-hold right on top of her areola with only her baby's mouth holding the nipple. Upon physical examination, the nurse finds that both her nipples and areolas are intact.

Assessment
During the assessment, the nurse collected the following data, which could be interpreted to be risk (causative/predisposing) factors for this diagnosis:
– Inappropriate maternal hand support of breast
– Inappropriate positioning of the infant during breastfeeding
– Use of products that remove the natural protection of the nipple

Although nurses cannot independently intervene upon at risk populations or associated conditions, it is important to be aware of individuals for whom a nursing diagnosis might be more likely to occur. Thus, the nurse should have identified the following at risk populations that would potentially alert the nurse to concerns for this diagnosis:
– Primiparous women
– Sole mother
– Women aged < 19 years

Listed below are some examples of nursing goals, outcomes and actions, linked to etiological factors. This is not presented as a comprehensive plan of care, but rather provides examples to demonstrate the proper method for linking diagnosis to outcomes and interventions, in an evidence-based manner.

D.Y.'s nursing diagnosis, ultimate goal, outcomes and nursing actions

Nursing diagnosis	Risk for nipple-areolar complex injury (00321)	
Ultimate goal(s)	Nipple-areolar complex integrity	
Risk factors	**Outcomes**	**Nursing actions**
Inappropriate maternal hand support of breast	Appropriate maternal hand support of breast	Teach use of appropriate maternal hand support of breast, with fingers behind the areola
Inappropriate positioning of the infant during breastfeeding	Appropriate positioning of the infant during breastfeeding	Teach use of appropriate infant positioning during breastfeeding
Use of products that remove the natural protection of the nipple	Does not use products that remove the natural protection of the nipple	Teach to apply expressed breast milk to nipple and areolar area to protect the skin

11. Safety/protection

Domain 11 • Class 2 • Diagnosis Code 00312

Adult pressure injury

T. Heather Herdman

NANDA International, Inc. Nursing Diagnoses: Definitions and Classification 2021–2023, 12th Edition, p. 495

Definition
Localized damage to the skin and/or underlying tissue of an adult, as a result of pressure, or pressure in combination with shear (European Pressure Ulcer Advisory Panel, 2019).

Model case
A.F. is an 89-year-old widow, living alone in an apartment. She is average weight for her age and gender, alert and oriented. Her only medical conditions are mild hypertension, which is well controlled on medication, and osteoarthritis. She has fallen twice in the past two months, with only minor injury, but has come to the clinic to see if there is anything she can do to prevent another fall. She indicates that she is becoming more afraid to walk, but she knows maintaining her mobility is critical to her long-term health.

She has a slight limp, and is favoring her left side, which she indicates is a result of her last fall, which occurred 5 days ago (x-ray examination was negative in the emergency room for a fracture). Since that time, she has significantly reduced her activity level, and is predominantly sitting throughout the day. During her examination, her skin and mucous membranes are noted to be dry, with some scaliness noted to the skin over her arms and legs. She admits that she is not drinking as much as normal because she has been limiting her walking back and forth from her chair to the kitchen. A 3.2 cm, shallow open ulcer with a pink wound bed is noted over her sacral area. She says the area is painful, but she had attributed it to her fall.

Assessment
During the assessment, the nurse collected the following data, which could be interpreted to be related (causative) factors for this diagnosis:
- Pressure over bony prominence
- Sustained mechanical load
- Decreased physical activity
- Decreased physical mobility
- Dehydration
- Dry skin
- Inadequate knowledge of pressure injury prevention strategies

11. Safety/protection

The nurse also collected the following data, which could be interpreted as a defining characteristics for this diagnosis:
- Pain at pressure points
- Partial thickness loss of dermis

Although nurses cannot independently intervene upon at risk populations or associated conditions, it is important to be aware of individuals for whom a nursing diagnosis might be more likely to occur. Thus, the nurse should have identified the following at risk population and associated condition that would potentially alert the nurse to concerns for this diagnosis:
- Older adults
- Cardiovascular diseases

Listed below are some examples of nursing goals, outcomes and actions, primarily linked to etiological factors. This is not presented as a comprehensive plan of care, but rather provides examples to demonstrate the proper method for linking diagnosis to outcomes and interventions, in an evidence-based manner.

A.F.'s nursing diagnosis, ultimate goal, outcomes and nursing actions

Nursing diagnosis	Adult pressure injury (00312)	
Ultimate goal(s)	Optimal tissue integrity	
Related factors	Outcomes	Nursing actions
Pressure over bony prominence Sustained mechanical load	Pressure reduction over bony prominences Minimize sustained mechanical load	Use a standardized, validated pressure injury classification system/tool to classify and document the level of tissue loss Reassess pressure injury at least weekly to monitor progress toward healing Apply hydrocolloid wound dressings Implement reactive air mattress or overlay Maintain head of bed as flat as possible Teach to adopt the 30° side lying position when positioning in bed
Decreased physical activity	Adequate physical activity	Assess current physical activity behaviors using the Frequency, Intensity, Type, Time (FITT) principle Initiate progressive competency-based exercise program
Decreased physical mobility	Adequate physical mobility	Conduct environmental assessment of the home using a standardized, validated tool Encourage self-directed behaviors focused on physical condition Perform directed-by-other mobility activities focused on physical condition

11. Safety/protection

Dehydration Dry skin	Adequate hydration	Assess hydration status at every visit using a standardized, validated tool Increase choice of beverages/fluid options Involve family and friends in hydration support Modify home environment where possible to support adequate hydration Provide increased opportunities to consume fluids
Inadequate knowledge of pressure injury prevention strategies	Adequate knowledge of pressure injury prevention strategies	Advise to perform regular offloading and repositioning as much as possible when spending prolonged periods sitting Encourage & teach to regularly reposition self when in bed and seated Implement a progressive seating schedule based on the response of the pressure injury and surrounding skin, and the individual's tolerance Implement repositioning reminder strategies to promote adherence to repositioning regimens
Defining characteristics	**Outcomes**	**Nursing actions**
Partial thickness loss of dermis	Optimal skin integrity	Teach and encourage to perform pressure relieving maneuvers
Pain at pressure points	Adequate pain management	Use non-pharmacologic pain management strategies as a first line strategy and adjuvant therapy Use principles of moist wound healing to reduce pressure injury pain

11. Safety/protection

Domain 11 • Class 2 • Diagnosis Code 00304

Risk for adult pressure injury

T. Heather Herdman

NANDA International, Inc. Nursing Diagnoses: Definitions and Classification 2021–2023, 12th Edition, p. 497

Definition
Susceptible to localized damage to the skin and/or underlying tissue of an adult, as a result of pressure, or pressure in combination with shear (European Pressure Ulcer Advisory Panel, 2019).

Model case
Mrs. M.J. is a 91-year-old widow, living at home with her daughter on hospice care with full time caregivers for support. She has a history of transient ischemic attacks, chronic obstructive pulmonary disease, multiple myeloma, history of complete lumbar disc deterioration with bone fusing, and bilateral peripheral neuropathy. She has experienced three major falls, which have led to a significant reduction in her mobility, primarily due to fear of falling. In the past six months, she has gone from being approximately 90% independent (needing assistance only for showering) to 75% dependent, needing support for all activities of daily living except for feeding herself. She requires assistance to transfer, walks only short distances (< 20 feet) using a walker with a one person assist or a wheelchair, and uses a handicapped shower with shower seat. She is using 2–3 L of oxygen continuously to maintain oxygen saturations ≥ 90 and for comfort with breathing. She has 2 + to 3 + pitting edema bilaterally in her lower extremities. She has intermittent periods of confusion, but generally is alert and oriented.

In the past year, she has lost nearly 60 pounds, has a body mass index of 16.1, and has little appetite. She has to be strongly encouraged to eat or drink anything other than coffee, and spends the majority of her time reading or napping in her recliner chair. She has no obvious body fat, and very prominent hip and spinal bones. She bruises easily, and her skin has frequent tears if she hits a body part on a hard surface. Due to her lack of muscle mass, she has difficulty moving in her chair and bed, and "scoots" quite a bit, causing friction. She has a Braden Scale score of 13, which indicates moderate risk for pressure injury.

Assessment
During the assessment, the nurse collected the following data, which could be interpreted to be risk (causative/predisposing) factors for this diagnosis:
- Increased magnitude of mechanical load
- Pressure over bony prominence

11. Safety/protection

- Shearing forces
- Surface friction
- Decreased physical activity
- Decreased physical mobility
- Dehydration
- Dry skin
- Protein-energy malnutrition

Although nurses cannot independently intervene upon at risk populations or associated conditions, it is important to be aware of individuals for whom a nursing diagnosis might be more likely to occur. Thus, the nurse should have identified the following at risk populations and associated conditions that would potentially alert the nurse to concerns for this diagnosis:

- Individuals receiving home-based care
- Individuals with body mass index below normal range for age and gender
- Older adults
- Cardiovascular diseases
- Edema
- Impaired circulation
- Medical devices
- Peripheral neuropathy

Listed below are some examples of nursing goals, outcomes and actions, linked to etiological factors. This is not presented as a comprehensive plan of care, but rather provides examples to demonstrate the proper method for linking diagnosis to outcomes and interventions, in an evidence-based manner.

M.J.'s nursing diagnosis, ultimate goal, outcomes and nursing actions

Nursing diagnosis	Risk for adult pressure injury (00304)	
Ultimate goal(s)	Optimal tissue integrity	
Risk factors	Outcomes	Nursing actions
Increased magnitude of mechanical load	Decrease magnitude of mechanical load	Use textiles with low friction coefficients
	Pressure reduction	Consider using a reactive air mattress or overlay
Pressure over bony prominences	over bony prominences	Determine repositioning frequency with consideration to the individual's level of activity and ability to independently reposition
Shearing forces	Minimize shearing forces	
Surface friction	Minimize friction	Teach caregivers to use the 30° side lying position when positioning in bed
		Maintain head of bed as flat as possible
		Promote seating out of bed in an appropriate chair or wheelchair for limited periods of time
		Minimize and redistribute pressure using dynamic weight shifting (tilt and recline)

11. Safety/protection

Decreased physical activity Decreased physical mobility	Adequate physical activity Adequate physical mobility	Assess current physical activity behaviors using the Frequency, Intensity, Type, Time (FITT) principle Conduct environmental assessment of the home using standardized, validated tool Consider a physical mobility protocol including progressive mobility and a nurse to advocate for and assist with client physical mobility Initiate progressive competency-based exercise program Encourage self-directed behaviors focused on physical condition Perform directed-by-other mobility activities focused on physical condition
Dehydration Dry skin	Adequate hydration	Assess hydration status at every visit using standardized scale Modify home environment where possible to support adequate hydration Increase choice of beverages/fluid options Provide increased opportunities to consume fluids Involve family and caregivers in hydration support Implement skin care regimen to include keeping skin clean and properly hydrated Implement a skin care regimen that avoids use of alkaline soaps and cleansers Implement a skin care regimen that protects the skin from moisture with a barrier product
Protein-energy mal-nutrition	Adequate protein-energy nutrition	Conduct a comprehensive nutrition assessment using standardized, validated instrument Adjust protein intake as needed Develop and implement an individualized nutrition care plan Offer high calorie, high protein fortified foods and/or nutritional supplements in addition to the usual diet

11. Safety/protection

Domain 11 • Class 2 • Diagnosis Code 00313

Child pressure injury

T. Heather Herdman

NANDA International, Inc. Nursing Diagnoses: Definitions and Classification 2021–2023, 12th Edition, p. 499

Definition
Localized damage to the skin and/or underlying tissue of a child or adolescent, as a result of pressure, or pressure in combination with shear (European Pressure Ulcer Advisory Panel, 2019).

Model case
A.Y. is an 11-year-old boy with severe spastic quadriplegia cerebral palsy. He suffers from seizures, and is incontinent of bladder and bowel. A.Y. requires full assistance for activities of daily living, and scores as a Level 5 on the Gross Motor Function Classification System (transported in a manual wheelchair). During his home health visit he is noted to have partial-thickness tissue loss on his left heel, with exposed dermis. Additionally, there is an area of non-blanchable erythema noted to intact skin on his coccyx, which is warmer than the adjacent skin. He seems to experience pain when this area is probed, although AY is nonverbal.

A.Y.'s father, a single parent, notes it is getting more difficult for him to completely lift him off the bed as he grows, and due to his spastic movements. His movements frequently change his position in the bed or chair, and his father notes that he knows this is causing friction as his position changes in the bed or chair, but he doesn't know how to lessen this.

Assessment
During the assessment, the nurse collected the following data, which could be interpreted to be related (causative) factors for this diagnosis:
– Altered microclimate between skin and supporting surface
– Difficulty for caregiver to lift client completely off bed
– Excessive moisture
– Inadequate access to appropriate equipment
– Pressure over bony prominence
– Shearing forces
– Surface friction
– Difficulty maintaining position in bed
– Difficulty maintaining position in chair
The nurse collected the following data, which would be interpreted as defining characteristics for this diagnosis:

- Localized heat in relation to surrounding tissue
- Pain at pressure points
- Partial thickness loss of dermis
- Purple localized area of discolored intact skin

Although nurses cannot independently intervene upon at risk populations or associated conditions, it is important to be aware of individuals for whom a nursing diagnosis might be more likely to occur. Thus, the nurse should have identified the following at risk populations that would potentially alert the nurse to concerns for this diagnosis:

- Children receiving home-based care
- Children with developmental issues

Listed below are some examples of nursing goals, outcomes and actions, primarily linked to etiological factors. This is not presented as a comprehensive plan of care, but rather provides examples to demonstrate the proper method for linking diagnosis to outcomes and interventions, in an evidence-based manner.

A.Y.'s nursing diagnosis, ultimate goal, outcomes and nursing actions

Nursing diagnosis	Child pressure injury (00313)	
Ultimate goal(s)	Optimal tissue integrity	
Related factors	Outcomes	Nursing actions
Altered microclimate between skin and supporting surface	Appropriate microclimate between skin and supportive surface	Keep skin clean and properly hydrated
		Cleanse skin promptly after episodes of incontinence
		Educate caregiver on importance of skin care regimen that includes cleansing the skin promptly after episodes of incontinence
Excessive moisture	Skin hygiene	Cleanse the pressure injury
		Cleanse the skin surrounding the pressure injury
		Avoid use of alkaline soaps and cleansers
		Protect skin from moisture with a barrier product
		Maintain areas of eschar undisturbed
Difficulty for caregiver to lift client completely off bed	Caregiver support for lifting child	Use appropriate mobilization techniques to avoid increased shear forces
Inadequate access to appropriate equipment	Optimal assistive device used for repositioning	Use moving and handling equipment manufactured from fabrics designed to reduce risk for pressure ulcers, when possible
		Identify community resources for accessing turning/transfer/lift equipment
		Identify community resources for caregiver support with child
		Support family in using assistive devices to promote bed and seated mobility

11. Safety/protection

141

Pressure over bony prominences	Pressure reduction over bony prominences	Select a uniform, consistent method for measuring pressure injury size and surface area
Shearing forces	Reduced shearing forces	Assess physical characteristics of wound bed, surrounding skin, and soft tissue at each pressure injury assessment
Surface friction	Reduced friction	Reassess at least weekly to monitor progress toward healing
		Educate the caregiver to monitor and document pressure injury healing progress
		Apply hydrocolloid, hydrogel, or polymeric membrane wound dressings
		Refer to a seating specialist for prolonged sitting in wheelchair
		Promote seating out of bed in an appropriate chair or wheelchair for limited periods of time
		Consider using a reactive air mattress or overlay
		Teach family to use 30° side lying position when positioning in bed
		Maintain head of bed as flat as possible
		Minimize and redistribute pressure using dynamic weight shifting (tilt and recline)
		Reposition individual to relieve or redistribute pressure using manual handling techniques and equipment that reduce friction and shear
		Elevate heels using a specifically designed heel suspension device or a pillow/foam cushion to offload heel completely
Difficulty maintaining position in bed	Maintains optimal position in bed	Reposition on an individualized schedule, unless contraindicated
Difficulty maintaining position in chair	Maintains optimal position in chair	If reclining is not appropriate or possible, ensure that the individual's feet are well-supported on the floor or on footrests when sitting upright in a chair or wheelchair
		Provide family with appropriate devices to support position in bed
Defining characteristics	**Outcomes**	**Nursing actions**
Pain at pressure	Adequate pain management	Use non-pharmacologic pain management strategies
		Use moist wound healing principles to reduce pressure injury pain points

Domain 11 • Class 2 • Diagnosis Code 00286

Risk for child pressure injury

T. Heather Herdman

NANDA International, Inc. Nursing Diagnoses: Definitions and Classification 2021–2023, 12th Edition, p. 501

> **Definition**
> Child or adolescent susceptible to localized damage to the skin and/or under-lying tissue, as a result of pressure, or pressure in combination with shear, which may compromise health (European Pressure Ulcer Advisory Panel, 2019).

Model case

P.G. is a 4-year old boy who broke both of his femurs in a bus accident. He had flexible rods placed bilaterally and is currently in a bilateral long leg hip spica cast. P.G. is overweight at 87.2 pounds (39.6 kg), and it is difficult for his mother to move him easily in bed. She has been unable to consistently turn him to a prone position, as she cannot afford caregiver support or equipment. It is summer and very warm, and the family has no air conditioning and only a small room fan. His mother says his linen is frequently damp from his perspiration, even though she uses only a light sheet to protect his privacy. He has also started to urinate in the bed at night, which had not been an issue prior to the accident. She notes that she does everything she can to keep the cast dry, and uses absorbent pads. She also has rolled cotton along the edge of the cast to keep it from irritating his skin.

P.G. complains that his lower torso and legs itch and he is desperate to scratch them. His mother says she has had to remove pencils and other items he has tried to use to scratch underneath the cast.

He scores as very high risk on the Glamorgan Pressure Injury Assessment Risk tool.

Assessment

During the assessment, the nurse collected the following data, which could be interpreted to be risk (causative/predisposing) factors for this diagnosis:

- Altered microclimate between skin and supporting surface
- Difficulty for caregiver to lift client completely off bed
- Excessive moisture
- Inadequate access to equipment for children with obesity
- Increased magnitude of mechanical load
- Pressure over bony prominence

- Shearing forces
- Surface friction
- Sustained mechanical load
- Use of linen with insufficient moisture wicking property
- Decreased physical mobility

Although nurses cannot independently intervene upon at risk populations or associated conditions, it is important to be aware of individuals for whom a nursing diagnosis might be more likely to occur. Thus, the nurse should have identified the following at risk populations and associated conditions that would potentially alert the nurse to concerns for this diagnosis:

- Children receiving home-based care
- Children with body mass index above normal range for age and gender
- Immobilization
- Medical devices
- Physical trauma

Listed below are some examples of nursing goals, outcomes and actions, linked to etiological factors. This is not presented as a comprehensive plan of care, but rather provides examples to demonstrate the proper method for linking diagnosis to outcomes and interventions, in an evidence-based manner.

P.G.'s nursing diagnosis, ultimate goal, outcomes and nursing actions

Nursing diagnosis	Risk for child pressure injury (00286)	
Ultimate goal(s)	Optimal tissue integrity	
Risk factors	**Outcomes**	**Nursing actions**
Altered microclimate between skin and supporting surface Excessive moisture	Appropriate microclimate between skin and supportive surface Appropriate skin moisture	Keep skin clean and properly hydrated Place incontinence pad across the genital area, tucking it under the front and back edges of the cast Ensure incontinence pad is changed any time it becomes wet Cleanse skin promptly after episodes of incontinence Educate caregiver on importance of maintaining skin clean and free of excess moisture Offer bedpan every 2–3 hours Avoid use of alkaline soaps and cleansers Protect skin from moisture with a barrier product Assess under the medical device for moisture Teach caregiver to use blow drier on low setting to keep skin dry under cast Assess skin under and around medical devices for signs of pressure related injury as part of routine skin assessment

Difficulty for caregiver to lift client completely off bed Inadequate access to equipment for children with obesity	Caregiver support for lifting child Caregiver support for turning child Adequate access to appropriate equipment	Identify community resources for accessing turning/transfer/lift equipment Identify community resources for caregiver support with child Use moving and handling equipment manufactured from fabrics designed to reduce risk for pressure ulcers, when possible Provide family with assistive devices to promote bed mobility
Increased magnitude of mechanical load Pressure over bony prominences Shearing forces Surface friction Sustained mechanical load	Reduced magnitude of mechanical load Pressure reduction over bony prominences Reduced shearing forces Reduced surface friction Reduced sustained mechanical load	Evaluate pressure injury risk using standardized, validated tool Reposition every 2–4 hours around the clock Avoid vigorously rubbing skin at risk of pressure injuries Cushion and protect skin at edge of cast with dressings or silicone pads Monitor for edema under medical device Educate client to inform family and care team of any discomfort Regularly seek self-assessment of comfort
Decreased physical mobility	Adequate physical mobility	Perform directed-by-other mobility activities focused on physical condition

11. Safety/protection

Domain 11 • Class 2 • Diagnosis Code 00287

Neonatal pressure injury

T. Heather Herdman

NANDA International, Inc. Nursing Diagnoses: Definitions and Classification 2021–2023, 12th Edition, p. 503

> **Definition**
> Localized damage to the skin and/or underlying tissue, as a result of pressure, or pressure in combination with shear, which may compromise health (European Pressure Ulcer Advisory Panel, 2019).

Model case

E.G. is a very unstable, very low birthweight 24-week gestational age infant with intrauterine growth retardation who has been in the neonatal intensive care unit for 17 days. She has been diagnosed with severe respiratory distress syndrome, septicemia, Grade III intraventricular hemorrhage, and pneumothorax. E.G. is currently ventilated with an endotracheal tube, has a peripherally inserted central catheter, nasogastric tube, and a chest tube. She also has 5-set ECG electrodes and pulse oximeter monitoring. Her warming table is covered with plastic wrap to maintain moisture for her skin.

Upon beginning her care, she is noted to have very moist skin, and her cap on her head is wet. After removal of the pulse oximeter from her right foot, a maroon colored, localized area of intact skin is noted on the top of the foot, and a shallow ulceration is noted to the bottom of the foot. There is also redness and localized heat noted at the chest tube insertion site. She scores as very high risk on the Glamorgan Pressure Injury Assessment Risk tool.

Assessment

During the assessment, the nurse collected the following data, which could be interpreted to be related (causative) factors for this diagnosis:
– Excessive moisture
– Pressure over bony prominence
– Shearing forces
– Surface friction
– Sustained mechanical load
– Decreased physical mobility
– Factors identified by standardized, validated screening tool
The nurse also collected the following data, which would be interpreted as defining characteristics for this diagnosis:
– Erythema

- Localized heat in relation to surrounding tissue
- Maroon localized area of discolored intact skin
- Skin ulceration

Although nurses cannot independently intervene upon at risk populations or associated conditions, it is important to be aware of individuals for whom a nursing diagnosis might be more likely to occur. Thus, the assessment identified the following at risk populations and associated conditions that would potentially alert the nurse to concerns for this diagnosis:

- Low birth weight infants
- Neonates < 32 weeks gestation
- Neonates experiencing prolonged intensive care unit stay
- Neonates in intensive care units
- Immature skin integrity
- Immature skin texture
- Immature stratum corneum
- Immobilization
- Medical devices
- Significant comorbidity

Listed below are some examples of nursing goals, outcomes and actions, primarily linked to etiological factors. This is not presented as a comprehensive plan of care, but rather provides examples to demonstrate the proper method for linking diagnosis to outcomes and interventions, in an evidence-based manner.

E.G.'s nursing diagnosis, ultimate goal, outcomes and nursing actions

Nursing diagnosis	Neonatal pressure injury (00287)	
Ultimate goal(s)	Optimal tissue integrity	
Related factors	**Outcomes**	**Nursing actions**
Excessive moisture	Appropriate skin moisture	Assess beneath medical device for moisture Cleanse skin promptly after episodes of incontinence Maintain skin clean and properly hydrated Protect skin from moisture with a barrier product
Pressure over bony prominences	Pressure reduction over bony prominences	Apply hydrocolloid wound dressings for noninfected Category/Stage II pressure injuries
Shearing forces	Reduced shearing forces	Assess vascular/perfusion status of the lower limbs, heels and feet at least once per day
Surface friction	Reduced friction	Avoid positioning neonate directly onto medical devices unless it cannot be avoided

Sustained mechanical load	Pressure reduction over bony prominences	Reduce or redistribute pressure at the skin-device interface by regularly rotating or repositioning the medical device and neonate Reduce or redistribute pressure at the skin-device interface by providing physical support for medical devices to minimize pressure and shear Regularly monitor tension of medical device securements Reposition neonate to relieve or redistribute pressure using manual handling techniques that reduce friction and shear Reposition neonate so that optimal off-loading of all bony prominences and to achieve maximum pressure redistribution Reposition using slow, gradual turns to allow time for stabilization of hemodynamic and oxygenation status every 2–3 hours, as tolerated Use textiles with low friction coefficients
Decreased physical mobility	Adequate physical mobility	Perform directed-by-other mobility activities focused on physical condition
Localized heat in relation to surrounding tissue	Normothermic skin	Maintain environmental temperature in thermoneutral zone
Defining characteristics	**Outcomes**	**Nursing actions**
Erythema Maroon localized area of discolored intact skin Skin ulceration	Optimal skin integrity	Assess the physical characteristics of the wound bed and the surrounding skin and soft tissue using a standardized, validated assessment tool at least once daily Assess skin under and around medical devices each shift Avoid use of alkaline soaps and cleansers Conduct age-appropriate nutritional screening and assessment Consider enteral or parenteral nutritional support

Domain 11 • Class 2 • Diagnosis Code 00288

Risk for neonatal pressure injury

T. Heather Herdman

NANDA International, Inc. Nursing Diagnoses: Definitions and Classification 2021–2023, 12th Edition, p. 505

Definition
Neonate susceptible to localized damage to the skin and/or underlying tissue, as a result of pressure, or pressure in combination with shear, which may compromise health (European Pressure Ulcer Advisory Panel, 2019).

Model case
R.H. is a very low birthweight 25-week gestational age infant, born in the last 18 hours. He was born via emergency Cesarean section due to severe bradycardia, and prolonged rupture of membranes (approximately 32 hours). His vitals are: HR 132, RR 38, T 36 degrees C / 96.8 degrees F (axillary), pO2 92%. He is ventilated with an orotracheal tube, and is receiving sedation. His temperature has dropped,, so plastic wrap has been used to maintain temperature on the warming table, with subsequent increase in moisture within that environment. He also has a temperature probe, pulse oximeter attached to his foot, and electrocardiogram patches. An umbilical line has been placed for fluids and medications. His modified Glamorgan Pressure Injury Assessment Tool score is 25, which places him at very high risk for pressure injury.

Assessment
During the assessment, the nurse collected the following data, which could be interpreted to be risk (causative/predisposing) factors for this diagnosis:
- Altered microclimate between skin and supporting surface
- Excessive moisture
- Pressure over bony prominence
- Decreased physical mobility
- Dehydration
- Water-electrolyte imbalance
- Factors identified by standardized, validated screening tool

Although nurses cannot independently intervene upon at risk populations or associated conditions, it is important to be aware of individuals for whom a nursing diagnosis might be more likely to occur. Thus, the nurse should have identified the following at risk populations and associated conditions that would potentially alert the nurse to concerns for this diagnosis:
- Low birth weight infants

- Neonates < 32 weeks gestation
- Neonates in intensive care units
- Immature skin integrity
- Immature skin texture
- Immature stratum corneum
- Immobilization
- Medical devices
- Pharmaceutical preparations

Listed below are some examples of nursing goals, outcomes and actions, linked to etiological factors. This is not presented as a comprehensive plan of care, but rather provides examples to demonstrate the proper method for linking diagnosis to outcomes and interventions, in an evidence-based manner.

R.H.'s nursing diagnosis, ultimate goal, outcomes and nursing actions

Nursing diagnosis	Risk for neonatal pressure injury (00288)	
Ultimate goal(s)	Optimal tissue integrity	
Risk factors	**Outcomes**	**Nursing actions**
Altered microclimate between skin and supporting surface Excessive moisture	Appropriate microclimate between skin and supportive surface Appropriate skin moisture	Keep skin clean and properly hydrated Avoid use of alkaline soaps and cleansers Protect the skin from moisture with a barrier product Cleanse skin promptly after episodes of incontinence Assess beneath medical devices for moisture Excessive moisture Appropriate skin moisture
Pressure over bony prominences	Pressure reduction over bony prominences	Ensure regular turning and repositioning regimen, with frequency of every 2–3 hours, if possible Assess relative benefits of using an alternating pressure air mattress Monitor tension of medical device securements with every care bundle (every 2–3 hours) Assess skin beneath and around medical devices
Decreased physical mobility	Adequate physical mobility	Perform directed-by-other mobility activities focused on physical condition
Dehydration	Adequate hydration	Assess hydration status at least once per shift Monitor daily weights Maintain environmental temperature in thermoneutral zone Use plastic shields/chambers/barriers and semipermeable membranes to prevent excess insensible water loss

Water-electrolyte imbalance	Water-electrolyte homeo-stasis	Monitor intake and output each shift, or more frequently if needed
		Monitor concentration of urine each shift
		Administer IV fluids as ordered
		Monitor electrolytes and consult with provider when out of normal range

Domain 11 • Class 3 • Diagnosis Code 00289

Risk for suicidal behavior

Girliani Silva de Sousa, Camila Takáo Lopes

NANDA International, Inc. Nursing Diagnoses: Definitions and Classification 2021–2023, 12th Edition, p. 528

> **Definition**
> Susceptible to self-injurious acts associated with some intent to die.

Model case

K.L. is a 17-year-old who was diagnosed with depression when he was 15 years old. He has been prescribed antidepressants and has been feeling hopeless due to difficulties in school. His parents wanted to enroll him in psychotherapy, but he refused to attend the appointments.

His parents discovered he had been cutting his upper thigh in the school bathroom and scheduled an appointment with the school principal, counselor, and nurse. During the meeting, K.L. reported that he feels lonely all the time after his boyfriend took his own life three months ago. He said they had romantic difficulties, so he feels extremely guilty for his death. He feels that he is not a valuable person anymore, and he did not feel that he could tell anyone else about how he felt because he was ashamed.

Assessment

During the assessment, the nurse collected the following data, which could be interpreted to be risk (causative/predisposing) factors for this diagnosis:
- Difficulty asking for help
- Difficulty coping with unsatisfactory performance
- Expresses loneliness
- Low self-esteem
- Reports excessive guilt
- Self-injurious behavior

Although nurses cannot independently intervene upon at risk populations or associated conditions, it is important to be aware of individuals for whom a nursing diagnosis might be more likely to occur. Thus, the nurse should have identified the following at risk populations and associated conditions that would potentially alert the nurse to concerns for this diagnosis:
- Adolescents
- Individuals with family history of suicide
- Depression

Listed below are some examples of nursing goals, outcomes and actions, linked to etiological factors. This is not presented as a comprehensive plan of care, but rather provides examples to demonstrate the proper method for linking diagnosis to outcomes and interventions, in an evidence-based manner.

K.L.'s nursing diagnosis, ultimate goal, outcomes and nursing actions

Nursing diagnosis	Risk for suicidal behaviors (00289)	
Ultimate goal(s)	Absence of suicidal behavior	
Risk factors	**Outcomes**	**Nursing actions**
Difficulty asking for help	Ability to ask for help	Use therapeutic communication techniques to discuss difficulty asking for help
Difficulty coping with unsatisfactory performance	Improved attention Satisfactory school performance	Use therapeutic communication techniques to discuss attention and memory Use therapeutic communication techniques to discuss perceived failure and quality of school performance
Expresses loneliness	Expresses feeling of belonging	Use therapeutic communication techniques to discuss habits Facilitate participation in groups of people with shared habits
Low self-esteem	Improved self-esteem	Encourage participation in groups that promote self-care Use therapeutic communication techniques to discuss and improve practice of exercise.
Reports excessive guilt	Ability to talk about feelings	Use therapeutic communication techniques to discuss current situation associated with guilt Use therapeutic communication techniques to discuss feelings about the future and plans for the future.
Self-injurious behavior	Absence of self-injurious behavior	Use therapeutic communication techniques to discuss psychological pain Use therapeutic communication techniques to discuss other behaviors to replace self-injurious behavior. Educate parents and school staff on vigilance of self-injurious objects and behaviors

11. Safety/protection

Domain 11 · Class 6 · Diagnosis Code 00280

Neonatal hypothermia

T. Heather Herdman

NANDA International, Inc. Nursing Diagnoses: Definitions and Classification 2021–2023, 12th Edition, p. 542

Definition
Core body temperature of an infant below the normal diurnal range.

Model case
Infant B.C., male, was born unexpectedly at approximately 3:30 this morning, in the elevator of her parents' apartment building as they were heading to the hospital. The elevator is on the outside of the building, and poorly heated. The temperature outside was approximately 32 degrees F / 0 degrees C. He arrived very quickly, taking both parents unaware, and the father noted it took less than 5 minutes for him to be born. The father hailed a cab and the infant arrived wrapped in his father's jacket, carried by his mother. The cab driver had radioed ahead to the hospital to notify them that a very small infant was en route, and a team was standing by with a heated isolette. Arrival at the hospital was at 3:58 this morning.

Infant B.C. is the fourth child for his mother, M.C., a 42-year-old G4P4. At approximately 3:00am she awoke and realized her water had broken. She was shocked, as she guessed she was about 28 weeks pregnant. She has had no prenatal care, lives with her three other children and her partner in a high rise tenement building, and says she had no transportation or health insurance to obtain medical care. M.C. and her spouse say that all other pregnancies were healthy and full term, and that they had home births with family supporting them in the deliveries. "My auntie has delivered dozens of babies in our neighborhood, and she delivered all of mine without any problems." The entire family appears somewhat malnourished, the other children are small for their ages, but they appear to be very close and supportive of one another.

Infant B.C. was aged at 29 weeks, weighed 1179 g, his Apgars were 3 on arrival to the emergency department and then 7 at 5 minutes after arrival. His axillary temperature was 95.8 degrees F / 34.4 degrees C. His blood glucose was 1.4 mmol/l. He was lethargic, with a heart rate of 64 on admission, and respiratory rate of 25–30 and in moderate respiratory distress. Cyanosis was present, and pO2 was 85%. Limbs were flaccid, cold to touch, face was slack in appearance. He was stabilized and transferred to the newborn intensive care unit.

Assessment

During the assessment, the nurse collected the following data, which could be interpreted to be related (causative) factors for this diagnosis:

- Delayed breastfeeding
- Excessive conductive heat transfer
- Excessive convective heat transfer
- Excessive evaporative heat transfer
- Excessive radiative heat transfer
- Inadequate caregiver knowledge of hypothermia prevention
- Malnutrition

The nurse also collected the following data, which would be interpreted as defining characteristics for this diagnosis:

- Acrocyanosis
- Bradycardia
- Decreased blood glucose level
- Hypoglycemia
- Hypoxia
- Increased oxygen demand
- Insufficient energy to maintain sucking
- Peripheral vasoconstriction
- Respiratory distress
- Skin cool to touch

Although nurses cannot independently intervene upon at risk populations or associated conditions, it is important to be aware of individuals for whom a nursing diagnosis might be more likely to occur. Thus, the nurse should have identified the following at risk populations and associated conditions that would potentially alert the nurse to concerns for this diagnosis:

- Low birth weight infants
- Neonates aged 0–28 days
- Neonates born by cesarean delivery
- Neonates born to an adolescent mother
- Neonates born to economically disadvantaged families
- Neonates exposed to low environmental temperatures
- Neonates with high-risk out of hospital birth
- Neonates with inadequate subcutaneous fat
- Neonates with increased body surface area to weight ratio
- Neonates with unplanned out-of-hospital birth
- Premature neonates
- Damage to hypothalamus
- Immature stratum corneum
- Increased pulmonary vascular resistance
- Ineffective vascular control
- Inefficient nonshivering thermogenesis
- Pharmaceutical preparations

Listed below are some examples of nursing goals, outcomes and actions, primarily linked to etiological factors. This is not presented as a comprehensive plan of

11. Safety/protection

care, but rather provides examples to demonstrate the proper method for linking diagnosis to outcomes and interventions, in an evidence-based manner.

B.C.'s nursing diagnosis, ultimate goal, outcomes and nursing actions

Nursing diagnosis	Neonatal hypothermia (00280)	
Ultimate goal(s)	Normothermia	
Related factors	**Outcomes**	**Nursing actions**
Delayed breastfeeding	Effective breastfeeding	Initiate breastfeeding as soon as possible Initiate skin-to-skin contact with mother Monitor blood glucose every 1–2 hours until stable Encourage frequent breastfeeding attempts of short duration if infant has insufficient energy to maintain sucking Supplement breastfeeding with feeding tube, if necessary, to maintain blood glucose
Excessive conductive heat transfer Excessive convective heat transfer Excessive evaporative heat transfer Excessive radiative heat transfer	Reduced heat transfer	Dry infant Use newborn cap to prevent evaporative heat transfer from head Initiate skin-to-skin contact with parent Maintain infant in climate controlled isolette/warming table, when not on parent's chest Monitor axillary temperature every 15 minutes until stable for at least 4 hours
Inadequate caregiver knowledge of hypothermia prevention	Caregiver knowledge of hypothermia prevention	Educate caregivers on methods of heat loss, and ensure they can verbalize understanding of dangers Educate caregivers on methods to manage thermoregulation in newborn, and ensure they can verbalize methods to promote and maintain normothermia Encourage skin-to-skin contact with parent Encourage breastfeeding
Malnutrition	Adequate nutrition	Consult nutrition services for evaluation of family nutrition Provide education on newborn nutritional needs

Defining characteristics	Outcomes	Nursing actions
Decreased blood glucose level	Normal blood glucose level	Monitor blood glucose every 1–2 hours until stable Supplement with dextrose orally or parenterally, as needed
Hypoxia Increased oxygen demand Respiratory distress	Normal oxygenation levels	Conserve oxygen needs by decreasing stimuli to infant, providing care in blocks every 3–4 hours, if possible Supplement with oxygen, as needed Monitor pO_2 until stable
Insufficient energy to maintain sucking	Preserve energy to support growth	Consider use of standardized tool to assess infant readiness for and tolerance of feeding, and to profile infant's developmental stage regarding specific feeding skills Conserve energy by decreasing stimuli to infant, as possible Observe infant for cues of stress during feeding Teach caregiver to observe infant cues of stress during feeding Allow for rest periods for reorganization of infant swallowing function Offer opportunities for deep breathing and brief resting periods while feeding Consider supplementing feedings using oral gastric tube until stable

11. Safety/protection

Domain 11 • Class 6 • Diagnosis Code 00282

Risk for neonatal hypothermia

T. Heather Herdman

NANDA International, Inc. Nursing Diagnoses: Definitions and Classification 2021–2023, 12th Edition, p. 544

Definition
Susceptibility of an infant to a core body temperature below the normal diurnal range, which may compromise health.

Model case
A.B. delivered a healthy baby girl, at term, through home birth with her midwife. A.B. is 16, unmarried, and her mother was present at the birth. A.B. plans to raise the child herself, and she lives with her mother in a small apartment. Immediately upon the midwife placing the infant on A.B.'s chest, her mother removed the infant from A.B.'s arms, and walked out into the lounge area of the apartment building, where other family members were present. A.B. had a major laceration requiring suturing, so the midwife was not able to immediately return the baby to A.B. for breastfeeding and skin-to-skin time. When the midwife is able to leave A.B., she finds the grandmother and her sister bathing the newborn in a bassinet that was prepared in the kitchen area of the lounge. Although it is quite warm, windows are open and an overhead fan is on in the kitchen.

Assessment
During the assessment, the nurse collected the following data, which could be interpreted to be risk (causative/predisposing) factors for this diagnosis:
- Delayed breastfeeding
- Early bathing of newborn
- Excessive evaporative heat transfer
- Inadequate caregiver knowledge of hypothermia prevention
Although nurses cannot independently intervene upon at risk populations or associated conditions, it is important to be aware of individuals for whom a nursing diagnosis might be more likely to occur. Thus, the nurse should have identified the following at risk populations and associated conditions that would potentially alert the nurse to concerns for this diagnosis:
- Neonates aged 0–28 days
- Neonates born to an adolescent mother
- Immature stratum corneum
- Inefficient nonshivering thermogenesis

Listed below are some examples of nursing goals, outcomes and actions, linked to etiological factors. This is not presented as a comprehensive plan of care, but rather provides examples to demonstrate the proper method for linking diagnosis to outcomes and interventions, in an evidence-based manner.

A.B.'s nursing diagnosis, ultimate goal, outcomes and nursing actions

Nursing diagnosis	Risk for neonatal hypothermia (00282)	
Ultimate goal(s)	Normothermia	
Risk factors	**Outcomes**	**Nursing actions**
Delayed breastfeeding	Effective breastfeeding	Initiate breastfeeding as soon as possible Monitor blood glucose every 1–2 hours until stable
Early bathing of newborn	Maintain newborn warm and dry	Dry infant Maintain skin-to-skin contact or dress in warm clothing/blankets
Excessive evaporative heat transfer	Reduced heat transfer	Use newborn cap to prevent evaporative heat transfer from head Initiate skin-to-skin contact with mother Swaddle infant in warm, dry blanket when not on parent's chest Monitor axillary temperature every 15 minutes until stable for at least 2 hours
Inadequate caregiver knowledge of hypothermia prevention	Caregiver knowledge of hypothermia prevention	Educate caregivers on importance of stable temperature prior to bathing Educate caregivers on methods of heat loss, and ensure they can verbalize understanding of dangers Educate caregivers on methods to manage thermoregulation in newborn, and ensure they can verbalize methods to promote and maintain normothermia

11. Safety/protection

Domain 13.
Growth/development

Class 2.   Development

Domain 13 • Class 2 • Diagnosis Code 00314

Delayed child development

T. Heather Herdman

NANDA International, Inc. Nursing Diagnoses: Definitions and Classification 2021–2023, 12th Edition, p. 568

> **Definition**
> Child who continually fails to achieve developmental milestones within the expected timeframe.

Model case

J.R. is six years old and has started first grade. He is at the 75th percentile for weight and the 80th for height. He is a friendly, smiling boy in his visit to the school nurse. His teacher, Mrs. Ross, has requested an evaluation because she believes that he has failed to achieve several normal developmental milestones. Mrs. Ross indicates that J.R. does not play well with other children because he won't follow rules or take turns, and he doesn't seem to sense when another child has been hurt or might be sad. She notes that he does not participate in conversation, other than to respond with one or two words, nor does he offer conversation unless it is solicited. However, he does smile a lot and is polite with adults.

Mrs. Ross notes that she has spoken to his parents during parent-teacher conferences, and they are in their mid-40 s, and explained to her that they had a laissez faire attitude toward parenting, believing a child should explore what he wants when he wants, and they shouldn't influence his learning or interests. They rarely interacted with J.R. during these conferences and, when they did, they spoke to him very much like an adult. His father indicated children must "make their own way in the world and learn to entertain themselves" rather than having adults cater to them. His mother said they taught him very early that "crying would not earn him extra attention", and that he needed to figure things out for himself. It was noted that J.R. didn't independently engage with his parents. When his parents would leave the conferences, Mrs. Ross had to encourage J.R. to join them, as they would simply leave the room without him. Even with encouragement, J.R. would very slowly walk out of the room, stopping to look at things, without any concern that his parents were already gone.

During his assessment, it is noted that J.R. does not seem to be able to spell any words, although he can sing the alphabet song. He also has problems counting beyond five and doesn't appear to recognize colors. After using the bathroom, it was apparent that he was not able to redress himself, although he did wash his hands. He was also unable to hold either a crayon or a pencil correctly and could only hold it in his fist. Although he seemed engaged, he wasn't able to catch even large soft balls very gently tossed to him, and his coordination is very awkward for his age.

Assessment
During the assessment, the nurse collected the following data, which could be interpreted to be related (causative) factors for this diagnosis:
Infant or Child Factors
- Inadequate attachment behavior
- Inadequate stimulation

Caregiver Factors
- Decreased emotional support availability

The nurse also collected the following data, which would be interpreted as defining characteristics for this diagnosis:
- Consistent difficulty performing cognitive skills typical of age group
- Consistent difficulty performing language skills typical of age group
- Consistent difficulty performing motor skills typical of age group
- Consistent difficulty performing psychosocial skills typical of age group

Although nurses cannot independently intervene upon at risk populations or associated conditions, it is important to be aware of individuals for whom a nursing diagnosis might be more likely to occur. Thus, the assessment identified the following at risk population that would potentially alert the nurse to concerns for this diagnosis:
- Children aged 0–9 years

Listed below are some examples of nursing goals, outcomes and actions, primarily linked to etiological factors. This is not presented as a comprehensive plan of care, but rather provides examples to demonstrate the proper method for linking diagnosis to outcomes and interventions, in an evidence-based manner.

J.R.'s nursing diagnosis, ultimate goal, outcomes and nursing actions

Nursing diagnosis	Delayed child development (00314)	
Ultimate goal(s)	Adequate child development	
Related factors	Outcomes	Nursing actions
Inadequate attachment behavior	Adequate attachment behavior	Assess quality of parent-child communication using a standardized, validated scale
		Assess quality of parent-child attachment using a standardized, validated scale
		Work with parents to address their accessibility and availability to the child
		Support caregivers in promptly identifying and responding to child cues, signals, behaviors, and needs
		Provide positive reinforcement of parenting skills
		Support caregivers in increasing sensitivity and responsiveness to child

13. Growth/development

Inadequate stimulation	Adequate stimulation	Encourage caregivers to stimulate child's exploration of his environment Encourage caregivers to follow the child's lead, help the child to focus, support child exploration, and scaffold development
Decreased emotional support availability	Adequate availability of emotional support	Encourage child to openly express emotions Encourage child to openly express needs Encourage parents to consistently respond to child's emotions Encourage parents to consistently respond to child's needs

Domain 13 • Class 2 • Diagnosis Code 00305

Risk for delayed child development

T. Heather Herdman

NANDA International, Inc. Nursing Diagnoses: Definitions and Classification 2021–2023, 12th Edition, p. 570

> **Definition**
> Child who is susceptible to failure to achieve developmental milestones within the expected timeframe, which may compromise health.

Model case
P.J. was born at 33 weeks to a 15-year-old single mother who did not realize she was pregnant until two weeks prior to birth, and therefore had no prenatal care; he was immediately placed for adoption. His mother was malnourished, homeless, and estranged from her own family members, who she indicated were abusive, and she felt she would be unable to provide care for him.

P.J. was in the 15th percentile for weight, 31st for length, and the 29th for head circumference at birth. He is now 8-months old and in foster care, in the 21st percentile for weight, 35th for length, and 31st for head circumference.

This is his third foster care placement since he was discharged. He was removed from the first placement due to an assessment of psychological neglect by the caregivers, along with possible malnutrition. The second placement was ended by the family because his behaviors included inconsolable crying, sleep pattern disturbance, and difficulty feeding. He exhibits minimal attachment behaviors, and his current foster parent indicates that almost any stimulation at all "sets him off", so she has been keeping stimulation to a minimum. She notes that he feeds better when she keeps stimulation lower, however she indicates that his constant crying has led to a lack of sleep and increased stress for her, and she is very anxious about how to care for him that is safe but that can lower her stress level.

Assessment
During the assessment, the nurse collected the following data, which could be interpreted to be risk (causative/predisposing) factors for this diagnosis:
Infant or Child Factors
– Inadequate attachment behavior
Caregiver Factors
– Anxiety
– Excessive stress

Although nurses cannot independently intervene upon at risk populations or associated conditions, it is important to be aware of individuals for whom a nursing diagnosis might be more likely to occur. Thus, the assessment identified the following at risk populations that would potentially alert the nurse to concerns for this diagnosis:
- Children aged 0–9 years
- Children born to economically disadvantaged families
- Children whose mothers had inadequate prenatal care
- Children with below normal growth standards for age and gender
- Low birth weight infants
- Premature infants

Listed below are some examples of nursing goals, outcomes and actions, linked to etiological factors. This is not presented as a comprehensive plan of care, but rather provides examples to demonstrate the proper method for linking diagnosis to outcomes and interventions, in an evidence-based manner.

P.J.'s nursing diagnosis, ultimate goal, outcomes and nursing actions

Nursing diagnosis	Risk for delayed child development (00305)	
Ultimate goal(s)	Adequate child development	
Risk factors	**Outcomes**	**Nursing actions**
Inadequate attachment behavior	Adequate attachment behavior	Educate caregiver about impact of adverse early life experiences on child's developmental problems regarding attachment behavior and stress regulation
		Assess quality of parent-child communication using a standardized, validated scale
		Assess quality of parent-child attachment using a standardized, validated scale
		Provide education to foster parenting skills and sensitive parenting
		Provide positive reinforcement of parenting skills
		Support caregiver in increasing sensitivity and responsiveness to child
Caregiver anxiety	Decreased caregiver anxiety	Consider remote/virtual follow-up management for caregiver
		Identify and provide information on support groups providing local or online support to individuals caring for preterm infants
		Educate caregiver in the use of relaxation techniques
		Encourage caregiver engagement in mindfulness practices

| Excessive stress in caregiver | Decreased caregiver stress | Educate on strategies for stress relief
Identify and provide information on support groups for individuals providing foster care for special needs children
Provide information on phone or virtual support services for caregivers of special needs children
Identify sources of respite care services |

Domain 13 • Class 2 • Diagnosis Code 00315

Delayed infant motor development

T. Heather Herdman

NANDA International, Inc. Nursing Diagnoses: Definitions and Classification 2021–2023, 12th Edition, p. 571

Definition
Individual who consistently fails to achieve developmental milestones related to the normal strengthening of bones, muscles and ability to move and touch one's surroundings.

Model case
Baby M.P. is eight months old, lives at home with his parents and three siblings. He was born via a normal vaginal delivery and was discharged home at 24 hours without any noted concerns. An adult uncle (F.A.) has just moved in with the family to try to offer some support with the children. They share a two bedroom apartment in a public housing building in the center of a large city. M.P.'s mother did not have prenatal care, nor has he had any well baby visits until today. His parents both work shift work in a factory, with his mother working evening shift and his father working night shift. His mother completed her 10th grade education and his father dropped out of school in his 11th year of education. The uncle is taking classes in business, works full time during the day, and stays with him during the time his mother and father are both at work. M.P.'s siblings are 3, 4, and 6 years old.

Uncle F.A. has brought M.P. in for his appointment today because his father is sleeping and his mother is on her way to work. He indicates it was his idea to bring M.P. in for evaluation because "he doesn't seem like a normal kid in the way he moves". He notes that M.P.'s parents don't spend a lot of time with him because they are busy taking care of the other kids, and they both work overtime whenever they can for the money. The oldest sibling was premature, spent months in the hospital, and has a lot of medical conditions, including partial blindness, problems with eating, and the uncle states,"he's mentally delayed, but a really happy boy". Uncle F.A. indicates the entire family is underweight, and that M.P.'s mother was malnourished before and during the pregnancy.

F.A. notes that M.P. spends most of his day in his crib in the living room, and only has one toy - a stuffed teddy bear. He also indicates that the family doesn't have enough to eat, although he does what he can to help them with food. He says the parents love their kids, but are exhausted and just don't have the energy to engage M.P. in play or in stimulating him. All of their caregiving time seems to be devoted to taking care of his oldest brother.

Upon evaluation, M.P. is in the 40th percentile for weight and height, and the 35th percentile for length. He has difficulty pushing himself up while prone. He does not appear to be able to roll from prone to supine positions. He also has difficulty remaining in an unsupported seated position, instead he tilts and then falls to his left side. When sitting supported, he leans heavily to his left side. Further, he does not have good head support when held in a supported standing position, or when seated without support. In both cases, his head bobs and then falls backwards, requiring support to bring it back to a neutral state. He can hold toys for a short period of time, but seems to have difficulty picking them up on his own. He appears to lack the initiative to attempt to roll or pick up objects, and when encouraged, he will only try one or two times and then he stops. He can bring his hands to his mouth. His social/emotional, anguage/communication, and cognitive milestones appear to be normal for his age. His eyes follow objects and people's faces, and he laughs and smiles.

Assessment
During the assessment, the nurse collected the following data, which could be interpreted to be related (causative) factors for this diagnosis:
Infant Factors
- Insufficient initiative
- Insufficient persistence

Caregiver Factors
- Does not encourage infant to grasp
- Does not encourage infant to reach
- Does not encourage sufficient infant play with other children
- Does not engage infant in games about body parts
- Does not teach movement words
- Insufficient fine motor toys for infant
- Insufficient gross motor toys for infant

The nurse also collected the following data, which would be interpreted as defining characteristics for this diagnosis:
- Difficulty maintaining head position
- Difficulty picking up blocks
- Difficulty rolling over
- Difficulty sitting without support

Although nurses cannot intervene upon populations who are at risk for a condition, or associated conditions, it is important to be aware of individuals for whom a nursing diagnosis might be more likely to occur. The assessment identified the following at risk populations that should alert the nurse to consider the possibility of this diagnosis:
- Boys
- Infants aged 0–12 months
- Infants born to economically disadvantaged families
- Infants born to large families
- Infants born to parents with low educational levels
- Infants living in home with inadequate physical space

13. Growth/development

- Infants whose mothers had inadequate antenatal diet
- Infants with below normal growth standards for age and gender

Listed below are some examples of nursing goals, outcomes and actions, primarily linked to etiological factors. This is not presented as a comprehensive plan of care, but rather provides examples to demonstrate the proper method for linking diagnosis to outcomes and interventions, in an evidence-based manner.

M.P.'s nursing diagnosis, ultimate goal, outcomes and nursing actions

Nursing diagnosis	Delayed infant motor development (00315)	
Ultimate goal(s)	Adequate infant motor development	
Related factors	**Outcomes**	**Nursing actions**
Insufficient initiative Insufficient persistence	Adequate infant motor development	Evaluate sensory processing with a standardized, validated tool Initiate caregiving interventions to support early child development in the first three years of life Use standardized, validated tool to assess infant motor development at 9-, 18-, and 30-month visits Implement tummy time and infant positioning to improve infant motor development Promote caregiver-infant dyad to promote responsive caregiver-infant interactions and strengthen caregiver-infant relationship
Does not encourage infant to grasp Does not encourage infant to reach Does not engage infant in games about body parts Does not teach movement words	Parents encourage infant motor development	Encourage caregivers to teach object control skills Enroll caregivers in early intervention program to improve infant motor development Initiate direct or indirect instructional strategies by providers to improve motor delay Encourage caregivers to provide infant with freedom to move Encourage caregivers to provide outdoor time for infant, when possible Support caregivers in promptly identifying and responding to infant cues, signals, behaviors, and needs Encourage caregivers to follow the infant's lead, help the infant to focus, support infant exploration, and scaffold development

Does not encourage sufficient infant play with other children Insufficient fine motor toys for infant Insufficient gross motor toys for infant	Adequate infant play	Encourage older children to interact with infant Offer toys/equipment to encourage fine motor skills Offer toys/equipment to encourage gross motor skills Promote learning and play materials, such as developmentally appropriate toys Provide in-home visiting program to improve caregiver knowledge of caregiving skills and early childhood development
Malnutrition	Adequate nutrition	Promote breastfeeding, if appropriate Provide nutrition education to caregivers Consider macronutrient or micronutrient supplementation, if needed

13. Growth/development

Domain 13 • Class 2 • Diagnosis Code 00316

Risk for delayed infant motor development

T. Heather Herdman

NANDA International, Inc. Nursing Diagnoses: Definitions and Classification 2021–2023, 12th Edition, p. 573

> **Definition**
> Individual susceptible to failure to achieve developmental milestones related to the normal strengthening of bones, muscles and ability to move and touch one's surroundings.

Model case

Infant A.P. was a very low birthweight preterm infant born at 26 weeks gestation, with APGAR scores of 4 and 6, who spent the first 12 weeks of life in a neonatal intensive care unit (NICU). She suffered from respiratory distress syndrome and was ventilated, had a Grade III intraventricular hemorrhage, unstable blood pressure, and her central line became infected, leading to sepsis. She experienced many episodes of oxygen desaturation and bradycardic events during her first six weeks of life. During her NICU stay her parents were incredibly attentive, with one or both of them in the unit around the clock.

After a long struggle, A.P. eventually was extubated, and graduated to a stepdown unit. She remained there primarily due to her inability to breast or bottle feed without significant desaturation events, and a very slow pattern of weight gain (< 10 g/day). She was discharged home with oxygen at 2 L via nasal cannula, and with tube feedings to supplement bottle feedings, at day 125 of life (nearly 18 weeks post-birth, or 4 weeks corrected age). Her growth charts showed her in the 20th percentile for weight and height, and the 25th percentile for head circumference at time of discharge.

When the home health nurse visits at two weeks post-discharge, she finds A.P. to be inexpressive. She does not seem to seek interaction, to interact with her environment, or to follow her parents' voices or attend to their faces. Plantar and palmar grasp is weak to absent, she displays minimal rooting, tonic neck and stepping reflexes. Moro reflex is normal. She does not appear to focus or follow an object (black and white toy) when moving it side to side, and her limbs are somewhat floppy and without tone. There are no toys visible in the home environment.

A.P.'s parents note that since discharge, one of them has carried her in a fabric wrap on their bodies at all times. She is maintained in this position except for diaper changes and bathing. The environment at home is kept fairly dark and very quiet, with parents whispering to one another and to A.P. Because she was very sensitive to noise and light when she was in the NICU, they keep her inter-actions to a minimum, as they fear she will become stressed. No one except the home health nurse and physical therapist is allowed to visit the home, because of their concerns about infection and overstimulation of A.P.

Assessment

During the assessment, the nurse collected the following data, which could be interpreted to be risk factors for this diagnosis:

Infant Factors
– Insufficient curiosity
– Insufficient initiative
– Insufficient persistence

Caregiver Factors
– Anxiety about infant care
– Carries infant in arms for excessive time
– Does not allow infant to choose toys
– Does not encourage infant to grasp
– Does not encourage infant to reach
– Does not encourage sufficient infant play with other children
– Insufficient fine motor toys for infant
– Insufficient gross motor toys for infant
– Limits infant experiences in the prone position

Although nurses cannot intervene upon populations who are at risk for a condi-tion, or associated conditions, it is important to be aware of individuals for whom a nursing diagnosis might be more likely to occur. The assessment identified the following at risk populations and associated conditions that should alert the nurse to consider the possibility of this diagnosis:
– Infants aged 0–12 months
– Infants in intensive care units
– Infants with below normal growth standards for age and gender
– Low birth weight infants
– Premature infants
– 5 minute APGAR score ≤ 7
– Neurodevelopmental disorders
– Postnatal infection of preterm infant

Listed below are some examples of nursing goals, outcomes and actions, linked to etiological factors. This is not presented as a comprehensive plan of care, but rather provides examples to demonstrate the proper method for linking diagno-sis to outcomes and interventions, in an evidence-based manner.

13. Growth/development

A.P.'s nursing diagnosis, ultimate goal, outcomes and nursing actions

Nursing diagnosis	Risk for delayed infant motor development (00315)	
Ultimate goal(s)	Adequate infant motor development	
Risk factors	Outcomes	Nursing actions
Anxiety about infant care	Reduced anxiety about infant care	Assess motor development using a standardized, validated assessment tool Allow parents to verbalize anxiety Refer to parenting support group for NICU parents Teach parents that a developmentally appropriate home environment and sensitive parent–infant relationship can positively impact the infant's ongoing learning experiences and development Teach parents that parent-delivered motor interventions should include active parental participation and implementation at regular intervals Teach parents that parent-delivered motor interventions should include an engaging environment
Carries infant in arms for excessive time Limits infant experiences in the prone position Does not encourage infant to grasp Does not encourage infant to reach	Adequate infant independent movement Adequate infant position changes Adequate encouragement of motor skills	Support midline positioning Support active infant movement Promote motor control through practice of infant-directed exploratory behaviors Teach parents to provide postural support Teach parents to provide opportunities for movement with support during parent–infant interaction Teach parents that parent-delivered motor interventions should include child-initiated active movements Consider massage therapy
Does not allow infant to choose toys Does not encourage sufficient infant play with other children Insufficient fine motor toys for infant Insufficient gross motor toys for infant	Adequate play exploration Appropriate use of toys to encourage fine motor development Appropriate use of toys to encourage gross motor development	Support play exploration Promote motor control through practice of infant-directed exploratory behaviors Teach parents to provide appropriate toys to encourage fine motor development Teach parents to provide appropriate toys to encourage gross motor development